YOUNG INNER CITY FAMILIES:
Development of Ego Strength Under Stress

YOUNG INNER CITY FAMILIES:
Development of Ego Strength Under Stress

Margaret Morgan Lawrence, M.D.

Behavioral Publications, Inc.
New York

Library of Congress Catalog Number 74-8153
ISBN: 0-87705-156-9
Copyright © 1975 by Behavioral Publications, Inc.

All rights reserved. No part of this work may be reproduced or utilized in any form or by any means, electronic or mechanical, including photocopying, microfilm and recording, or by any information storage and retrieval system without permission in writing from the publisher.

BEHAVIORAL PUBLICATIONS, INC.
72 Fifth Avenue
New York, New York 10011

Printed in the United States of America
56789   987654321

Library of Congress Cataloging in Publication Data

Lawrence, Margaret Morgan, 1914–
   Young inner city families.

   Includes bibliographical references.
   1. Child mental health—New York (City)   2. Poverty—Psychological aspects.   I. Title.   [DNLM: 1. Child   psychiatry. 2. Ego. 3. Negroes. 4. Stress, Psychological. WS350 L422y 1974]
RJ111.L33   618.9'28'905   74-8153

But ours is a subtle strength
Potent with centuries of yearning,
Of being kegged and shut away
In dark forgotten places.

> from, "To the Oppressors" in *Dark Testament and Other Poems* by Pauli Murray, Norwalk, Silvermine, 1970

Contents

	Introduction	7
I.	Nature, Nurture and Noxia in a Black Community	21
II.	Nature	36
III.	Nurture	55
IV.	Noxia	69
V.	Hasson: A Brief Multi-Agency Study	81
VI.	Pedro: A Harlem Child Study By Frances Gautieri Ricigliano, A.C.S.W.; Helen R. Drew, B.S.; Irene J. Spanier, M.S.; Margaret Morgan Lawrence, M.D.; and Katrina de Hirsch, F.C.S.T.	97
VII.	Mission	130
	References	137

Introduction

Young inner city families, for the most part black and Hispanic, bring their infants and preschool children to the doors of various child-caring agencies in the Harlem Hospital Center community in New York City. This volume describes these young families from the viewpoint of a child psychiatrist and devoted member of a mental health team. The vignettes painted here from child health station, Developmental Psychiatry Clinic, Therapeutic Nursery and day care center also take on my personal perspective: that of my history, my cultural background, my family including my extended family and the communities in which I was reared. These in turn contribute to mind, body and "soul," a "self" that has been freely used in the dramas or plays of which these vignettes are accurate representations.

It is not difficult to find myself, a black, identified with poor, black, needy people. I share history, culture, communities with them. I live, however, on a social class and economic level somewhat different from that of many of the families with whom I work, although ofttimes their relatives or families down South share my relative affluence. Nevertheless, I share the conviction that, regardless of social and economic class, they and I have identical goals and dreams for our children. It is true, however, that my middle-class status and comparative affluence have protected me from many of the stresses of body, nurture and frank trauma to which they have been subjected. In spite of these overwhelming stresses which tend to discourage involvement with poor families, some knowledge of my own ego strength is an aid to recognition of theirs, and awareness of my own neurotic conflicts gives me empathy with theirs. This book speaks of our common humanity, intends to indicate opportunities for emotional re-education and points the way to revival of ego strengths among a large population of the urban poor.

The making of this psychoanalytically oriented community child psychiatrist was accomplished in an academic world that was largely white. Well identified with the black world from the days of my childhood, I was never alien to the white world. The latter paid my father's salary, educated me through most of high school, college, medical and psychiatric training. It might be said that I have lived and have been educated in two worlds. From the perspective of these two worlds made one in my own life and history, the distance is spanned from therapy, even psychoanalysis, in the consultation room or playroom, to consultation to the staff of a day care center. In both settings I find it important to estimate the ego strength of the persons with whom I intend to collaborate. I can then lend my tools, including myself as a principal tool, for the reconstruction and reintegration of their strengths. The story of the development of this principal tool may lend credence to my part in the dramas that follow.

My life history is not a tale of rags to riches, nor even the story of a journey from ghetto to the academic ranks of a white institution. I am the daughter of a very middle-class teacher and Episcopal priest, and the grandniece of an early-twentieth-century Virginia teacher. In the Mississippi community in which I grew up, I played with my small friends beside their mother's chair, in the same room where their uncle was "laid out" in his coffin. With the same friends I shared the "mourners' bench" in the Baptist Church when, in our adolescence, revival time came, for my father was an active ecumenicist long before the word "ecumenical" became fashionable.

The distance does not seem far between the rural Thanksgiving table, groaning with food, provided by a "grass widow" member of my father's church and made elegant by her admonition to one of her sons, "Brother, take your elbows off the table," to the conference room in a psychiatric institute devoted to research. When I heard there that a ten-year-old black boy and his mother were not suitable for psychodynamic psychotherapy, and that recourse had to be taken, in our despair, to "supportive measures," my mind began to drift to one of these older rooms in my own history.

In crises of death, adolescence, or when a husband ran away, the black people I knew in the urban and rural Mississippi of fifty years ago turned to religion for comfort in the literal sense of the word; that is, through religion they "joined" their strength, body, mind and soul: "You took my feet out of the mire-y clay and placed them on a firm foundation." Each individual, man or woman, boy or girl, became the "tool" of his own reconstruction. "Soul" was a matter of depth of being, as compared with more superficial feelings or emotions; although these more superficial expressions of feeling accompanied the deeper sense of "soul." Expression of soul was free, and was further enhanced in community.

These are memories from home in Mississippi. But to recapitulate, throughout my life I have felt that I never wholly left Harlem after the age of three. I was born in New York, but not in Harlem. Negroes in 1914 lived, among other places, in the West 60's, and my mother had come there to have her baby. Grandma had arrived in the West 60's not long before, from Richmond, Virginia. I was not born in Harlem Hospital, where my first child was born, but in Sloane's Hospital for Women, which later moved to Columbia-Presbyterian Medical Center. I went to medical school there in 1936.

Some years later, my aunt took a picture of Grandma and me on 137th Street between Lenox and Fifth Avenues. She shot the photograph from the apartment window, and one could hardly tell that there were two people, one very large and one rather small. Harlem Hospital loomed up behind us. It looked very big. Grandma moved to 137th Street because it was a good neighborhood, and not too expensive. Two years later, when my mother and I made our biennial trip to Grandmother's, dressed in the browns and navy blues made for us by Mrs. McCraven, our dressmaker in Vicksburg, Mississippi, Grandma had moved to a swankier neighborhood on Seventh Avenue and 141st Street. There was a park with nice green plantings in the middle between the uptown and downtown sides of the street. Parades passed nearly every Sunday. In those days, nearly all of Grandma's friends went to Harlem Hospital when they were sick, and called the ambulance freely. At the time of that particular trip, my mother, father and I had just moved to Vicksburg from Mount Bayou, an all-Negro town of about 2,000 souls in Mississippi's delta. Vicksburg, a hilly city, famous for its Civil War battles, then had a population of about 20,000. My mother took these moves badly.

Shortly after we arrived in Vicksburg, Mother and I took a vacation in New York in Grandma's new apartment. I was enrolled for a month in the kindergarten around the corner. There, children said "Good morning," in concert, to the principal, and played with beads. I had learned to read two years earlier in Widewater, Virginia, in a school in the rural church where my mother taught. Aunt Hazel, my mother's sister, no longer lived with Grandmother. She had married and "opened up," that is, desegregated, a house on "Sugar Hill." They hadn't known she was a Negro. I think that the members of my family were the only people in Vicksburg, colored or white, who took vacations every two years in New York. Most people went to Chicago. That is what the railroad man, the father of my redheaded friend who lived next door said when he got us our long tickets. He was white.

History, in fact and in symbol, contains the germ of the future. In my own lifetime, I walked across the street from my childhood Mississippi home again and again to hear the story of a doctor-husband tarred and feathered and run out of town because he dared to treat white patients. Years later, in Washington Heights, Manhattan, while a medical student at Columbia Medical Center, intending to vote for the first time for a president of the United States, I had to take a "litaracy test." I framed that certificate of literacy. On the same streets I had several offers of "day work." I have been denied a pediatric interneship at the medical center from which I graduated as a physician, and was welcome to a pediatric fellowship in the same institution seven years later, when the racial climate in the city and nation had markedly changed. I was a "first" at New York State Psychiatric Institute and Columbia Psychoanalytic Clinic, caught in the wake of the humanizing post-World War II waves which dashed on a neutral-colored bedrock that included Quakers, psychiatrists and psychoanalysts, and journalists.

The year 1940 that marked my graduation from medical school and the refusal of a pediatric interneship, both at Columbia Medical Center, was also marked by my introduction to a great physician, Louis T. Wright, M.D., a black man, then Medical Director of Harlem Hospital. At the time of the comprehensive competitive examinations that preceded our selection as internes and residents at Harlem Hospital, fellow applicants were chiefly persons of Jewish and Italian backgrounds, a very talented group. When I began my own two-year rotating interneship on July 1, 1940, I discovered that the discrimination which had operated against young Jewish, Italian and a small number of Negro doctors seeking further medical training, as well as against the senior physicians who comprised the hospital's attending staff, had also operated to provide Harlem with a house staff and a visiting staff of high calibre. We were all free, however, as is the youth of our time, to express openly the ideals of our recent adolescence; ideals, I had occasion to discover, which were often identical with those of many of our middle-aged and elderly medical mentors. We appeared in uniform before New York City's Board of Estimate, asking for needed medicines and materials for our Harlem Hospital. We were also protesting the fact that medical internes received a salary of only $18.00 a month, and we asked for an increase.

Following my interneship at Harlem, there was a year's pause, significant because it tapped for me a latent sense of "mission" that had been part of the history of my family, and my husband's family as well. I spent the year 1942–43 at what was then called the Columbia School of Public Health. Harry Stoll Mustard and Haven Emerson were among my teachers. The germ, however, of what might be called community child mental health was planted for good during months in a seminar led by Dr. Benjamin Spock at the Kips Bay–Yorkville Child Health

Station. His exciting and well-integrated vision of the child, the family, the community and society never left me. In May, 1943, our first child was born at Harlem Hospital. Twenty years passed before I again returned to Harlem Hospital.

In September, 1943, with World War II very much a part of our lives, our family moved to Nashville, Tennessee. My husband taught sociology at Fisk University and joined the Race Relations Institute, and I taught pediatrics and public health, separately and in combination, at Meharry Medical College. Four years later we left Nashville to return to New York City and further study. Both adults had fellowships. Our family had increased to five.

In 1946, Clarence Pickett of the American Friends Service Committee introduced me to Viola Bernard, later founder and Director of Columbia University's Division of Community and Social Psychiatry. She was able to draw for me a picture of psychoanalytic community child psychiatry which was indeed relevant to my own life history and dreams. She has not relented from pressing for that ideal image, whether in the planning and education phase of community mental health services in Rockland County, or in our various mental health functions in New York City.

The years from 1947 to 1951 included a memorable year in pediatrics with Hattie Alexander, M.D. at Babies Hospital; my personal analysis with Eugene Milch, M.D.; a psychiatric residency at the New York State Psychiatric Institute while Nolan D. C. Lewis, M.D. was Director; and training in the Columbia Psychoanalytic Clinic for Training and Research directed by Sandor Rado, M.D. Wide-eyed, I was witness to Dr. Rado's "massive-dose" direct therapy, freely given in the midst of a case conference. Dr. Lewis taught me that a brain-injured child can himself affect the attitudes and behavior of his mother. It was my great privilege to have David Levy and Nathan Ackerman as supervisors in child therapy, the latter during a child psychiatric residency at the therapeutic nursery of the Jewish Board of Guardians; the nursery was then called the Council Child Development Center, and I was their pediatric consultant. It was at this Center that I was given the opportunity to join with Peter Neubauer, M.D., Samuel Ritvo, M.D., and others of a multidisciplinary child mental health team, in organizing and functioning in a consultation unit to day care centers. This ended the period of my formal psychiatric training.

My next 12 years were spent in Manhattan and Rockland County, New York. I organized and participated in consultation units to neighborhood day care centers at the Northside Child Development Center with Mamie Clark, Ph.D., its Director, Olivia Edwards, M.S.W., psychiatric social worker, and others. Later, at the Educational Clinic of the City College of New York, Florine Katz, Ph.D., and I, together with others in a multidisciplinary educational and mental health team, increased our awareness of the role of organicity in emotional and learning problems. We set up consultation services to day care centers and one public school, and initiated child-study groups with student teachers. In Rockland County, New York, where our family had made its home in 1951, I participated in the planning, organization and community education for community mental health services in the county with a host of other mental health workers. Also, with John A. P. Millet, M.D., I co-directed the Community Mental Health Center, which operated on a voluntary basis for one year. With Louis C. English, M.D., as Director of the Community Mental Health Board and the Community Mental Health Center, I was Associate Director in charge of Children's Services from 1954 to 1957, and from the latter year until 1963, I was Director of the School Mental Health Unit, a consultation service to the schools of Rockland County. The unit's other stalwart team members were Mildred W. Dubowy, M.S.W., and Irene J. Spanier, M.S., clinical psychologist. A record of this enterprise is to be found in *Mental Health Team in the Schools* written by this author. Overlapping the termination of the School Mental Health Unit and my return to Harlem was the organization of, and my own part in the life of, the Day Treatment Center of the Rockland County Organization for Mentally Ill Children. Mrs. Jean W. Houser was the Treatment Center's Educational Director. It was there that the significance of the intertwining of history, nature, nurture and trauma became most obvious. By the light of ideas that reached our consciousness as early as 1962, we were able to draw our first sketches of a comprehensive early childhood development center for our county. Seven years later these ideas came to fruition in a Child Development Center for infants and children under the age of five. This Center is a unit of the comprehensive Rockland County Community Mental Health Center of the Rockland Health Complex. Timothy Moritz, M.D., and Martin Hart, M.D., became, respectively, Director of the Mental Health Center and Director of the Division of Children and Youth of that Center.

I returned to Harlem Hospital in 1963. Their Department of Psychiatry had become affiliated in 1962 with the Department of Psychiatry of Columbia University's College of Physicians and Surgeons. At the Harlem Hospital Center, Elizabeth Davis, M.D., was Director of the Department of Psychiatry, and Virginia Wilking, M.D., directed its Division of Child Psychiatry. Drs. Davis and Wilking gave me free rein to plan and organize a Developmental Psychiatry Unit of the Division of Child Psychiatry with them and others of their multidisciplinary staff, notably Miss Kathleen Goodin, chief psychiatric social worker of the Division of Child Psychiatry, and Cesarina Paoli, M.D., child psychiatrist, organizer of the Division's Therapeutic Nursery. I believed and contributed to the statement made in *Crisis in Child Mental Health*, "Challenge for the 1970's," the report of the Joint Commission on Mental Health of Children:

> Poverty, in this the richest of world powers, is still our heritage. Racism, in a country dedicated to its people's inalienable rights, speaks as clearly of 'man's inhumanity to man' as did slavery [p. 1].

As vice-chairman of the Subcommittee on Problems and Priorities of the New York State Committee for Children from its initiation in May, 1971, I chaired a Task Force on Early Childhood which reported to Governor Nelson A. Rockefeller (1971) that "prevention and developmental needs" are among areas of major concern, that

> the period of infancy and early childhood [including the prenatal and paranatal periods] is crucial in the development of good health and adaptive behavior

and that

> [a] Child Advocacy Commission would need to give emphasis to the promotion of pilot efforts in comprehensive early childhood development centers. Federal legislation now being considered in Congress which would support the development of comprehensive day care centers is a step in this direction, especially if it results in more effective integration of all community services on behalf of infants and preschool children [pp. 22–23].

The bill that would have resulted in the Comprehensive Child Development Act of 1971 was vetoed by President Nixon, almost as the Report of the Committee for Children was submitted to the governor. It would have offered support to families in providing settings, human contacts and care designed for the optimal development of children. Today, in 1974, such hopes are even more distant.

The parables in the book that follows, true vignettes of well-baby station, Developmental Psychiatry Clinic, Therapeutic Nursery, and day care center, are told in the context of Harlem Hospital Center. Most of the actors are black, and those workers who are not "could pass." During the past 30 years the scene has changed at Harlem Hospital Center and the institution to which it is affiliated, Columbia University College of Physicians and Surgeons; but whether "in the bottoms" or "on the hill," the legacy of poverty, racism and dehumanization still plagues us. We are still, black and white, too little aware of the inherent and historical strengths of those with whom we labor. And the tools of our various disciplines are made dull in our own despair. We have tried everything that we know, and we say it does not work. We defend ourselves for our lack of success with the belief that our precious tools, such as psychiatry, even community psychiatry, and psychoanalysis do not apply for the poor and the minorities in our population.

I call upon those engaged in work on the hills and in the bottoms of our land to join in using their disciplines and themselves as tools to bring into relief our own strengths and resources of body, mind and soul, current and historical, and the strengths and resources of the people with whom we work. The parables that follow, a few unorthodox, but perhaps not new, demonstrate ways in which these tools may be used. At Harlem Hospital Center the procedures outlined here have been short in duration, often out spoken and dramatic, full of action, looking for opportunities, high in zeal and expectation, and trusting of co-workers both colleagues and young families.

John Spiegel (1973) in a position paper concerning his "stand on issues important to the profession of psychiatry in the 1970's," written prior to his election to the presidency of the American Psychiatric Association, states:

> In their training I believe that students and residents should be taught to utilize the biological and psychodynamic principles traditional to psychiatry as well as the newer therapies and be able to place all of them within an historical perspective. But, they should also learn to see mental health care through the eyes of the collaborating professions: other physicians, nurses, psychologists, social workers, sociologists, paraprofessionals and of various socio-economic classes and regional or subcultural groupings of consumers. In other words, citizens wanting or needing our services should not be seen as "targets" at which we aim our expertise, but as collaborators in the maintenance or restoration of health [p. 3].

I wish that this statement, which is directed specifically to psychiatrists, might be found worthy, by our collaborators, to enjoin us all to our mutual responsibility. I find it relevant to the purpose of the parables which follow.

I

NATURE, NURTURE AND NOXIA IN A BLACK COMMUNITY

> It is remarkable that blacks have survived and increased in numbers. They have had to learn, in the service of survival, to be able to listen to, *tune in,* and *turn off* unconscious racism (not to mention its conscious variety). It is remarkable that their own deep-rooted human insecurities of impermanence have not been potentiated by the added crippling affects associated with living from day to day in a dehumanizingly cruel racist environment. In a less stouthearted group, extinction would likely have been their fate. Their past adaptational defenses, patience and hope, have coalesced and resulted in an increasingly tougher and rugged character structure, as we are now witness to [Prudhomme, 1970, p. 816].

In a workshop on Psychoanalysis and Community Mental Health held in December 1968, members of the American Academy of Psychoanalysis inquired of their responsibility in antipoverty programs. They concluded

> that there is need to identify and use the strengths found among the various poor, in

their lives and in their community institutions. While it is important to identify a community's leaders and to find out what the people want, psychoanalysts and other mental health workers must recognize what they themselves have to offer, based in their own disciplines, in collaboration with the people whom they wish to serve.

I, too, am among an increasingly large number of psychoanalysts and other mental health workers who recognize and feel challenged by the ego strengths of the poor, blacks and other minorities—strengths that have survived great stress. Many psychoanalysts, traditionally tied to their ivory towers—an easy chair at the head of a couch—have found important roles to play in the sprawling new edifices of community psychiatry. They share their discipline with those of others in mental health teams, and test their understanding of the dynamics of human development against other hypotheses. They must work with a less manageable population than that to be found in their private consultation rooms, but through this population, transcultural experiences bring greater wisdom and new insights. These analysts expose themselves and their strengths to a shared humanity in people less fortunate, socially and economically, than themselves. They discover ego strengths that have survived terrible odds, and depth of feeling beneath sullen faces.

Within a span of 24 years, I have twice served children in the Harlem Hospital community. My decision, in 1940, after four years in medical school, to get the best possible training in pediatrics, led me to apply first for a pediatric interneship at Babies Hospital, Columbia Medical Center. Pediatric training at Harlem Hospital was a second choice; however, this experience provided excellent training in the physical care of infants and children, and certainly led to my return years later with additional familial, social and historical concerns. These concerns, in turn, were prompted by my own personal history. They came from the intervening years of training and experience in public health, pediatrics, and child health in a southern black medical school and community; in psychiatry, child psychiatry, psychoanalysis, mental health consultation projects for schools and centers for young children; and in the study of developmental disabilities.

The story that follows began at Harlem Hospital Center upon my return in 1963. It is the story of a committed interdisciplinary mental health team, black and white, who search out the ego strengths of young Harlem families, in the hospital, on the streets, in the child care centers and health facilities; wherever young children, particularly those who present problems in growing and developing, are to be found. This team is the Developmental Psychiatry Unit team of the Division of Child Psychiatry in the Department of Psychiatry, Harlem Hospital Center. The Developmental Psychiatry Unit's team includes a clinical psychologist, two psychiatric social workers, a psychiatric nurse, three part-time psychiatrists and three teachers. One teacher is the educational director of our Therapeutic Nursery and our educational consultant; and one other is a fully-trained early childhood teacher. The third, an assistant or teacher-aide, and a transportation aide, began their training in a community "self-help team." They have continued their training for the past three years by participating in the program of the Developmental Psychiatry Unit.

While the Developmental Unit serves infants and children under five years of age and their families, other units in the Division of Child Psychiatry respond to the needs of five-to-twelve-year olds, and adolescents. With a clear emphasis on the ego strengths of the families with whom they work, the Developmental Psychiatry Unit must search out and respond to those infants and young children in the community who present developmental, including emotional, problems, assessing their problems and strengths, and providing treatment, especially therapeutic education, for them and their families. The outreach program for this age group is equally important. The Unit collaborates with other child-care agencies such as day care centers and child health stations, their educators and counselors, their public health nurses, physicians and social workers. This outreach program, that is, mental health consultation to other agencies, not only provides access to the Developmental Psychiatry Unit for the children and families in the Harlem community which it serves; it assists these professionals in the use of their skills and facilities within their own setting. Consultation helps them in the recognition and management of minor problems, similar to the more severe ones that occur in children referred for evaluation by the Unit team. Consultation also supports workers in the recognition of children's assets, and possible paths to optimal development.

Child health stations, also called well-baby clinics, were being conducted by the City's Health Department throughout New York City, for all infants and preschool children who applied, when I arrived for my interneship at Harlem Hospital in 1940. These child health stations offered preventive care during a child's first five years, chiefly developmental examinations and immunization against communicable diseases. As of 1970, they were still being conducted in this form. With the 1970 merger of the city's departments of Health and Hospitals into a Health and Hospitals Corporation, many child health stations maintain much of their original form but are also closely related to city hospital departments of pediatrics. More easily than in the past, they can associate preventive with treatment measures. The Developmental Unit of the Division of Child Psychiatry anticipated the closer connection between hospitals and child health stations by providing bimonthly mental health consultation to each of five Harlem well-baby clinics. This experience, as it occurred until three to four years ago, and now somewhat altered by changes in child-health-station structure and the participation of other city hospitals with them, will be briefly described here.

A Developmental Unit team, in this case a psychiatric nurse and a child psychiatrist, and child health station physicians, nurses, social workers, and clerks, met in a circle with a child or children, his parents, and sometimes members of his extended family. This meeting occurred in a building constructed for the well-baby clinic, a housing development, or a Health Department district office building. The nurse-in-charge, who regularly assigned infants and children to "well-baby conferences," limited the number of these on the assigned morning in order to accommodate consultations of at least one-and-one-quarter hours each, concerning not more than two children. Not infrequently, trauma was the subject of a well-baby conference consultation. When a grandmother brought a three-year-old girl to the conference complaining of her withdrawn behavior, she told us that the little girl's mother had been fatally wounded when she was hit by a car several months before. Catharsis for the event, that is, the opportunity for open expression of feeling, together with identification of strength to sustain them in the face of such severe emotional trauma, was provided for both the child and the grandmother. Follow-up visits with this family in their home were arranged by a participating nurse to repeat this procedure. Referral to the Developmental Psychiatry Clinic was made for further evaluation and brief therapy. Within several therapeutic sessions, the little girl became much less withdrawn. Because of her needs and those of her physically-ill grandmother, she was then enrolled in a day care center.

The public health nurse-in-charge of the child health station conferred with our psychiatric nurse on how to refer a child and his family to the Developmental Psychiatry Unit within the hospital. Often the public health nurse would sit by a mother as she telephoned the Unit social worker to make her first hospital contact. During the next several days, the Unit social worker, in turn, made additional calls to arrange for an appointment with, and guided the parent and child to, a Pediatric Developmental Screening Clinic located in the Department of Pediatrics of Harlem Hospital. During this appointment the child's and family's needs were further appraised, and the most appropriate hospital clinic or clinics to serve these needs were determined. The Screening Clinic for preschool children met every two weeks for an afternoon, and was composed of pediatricians, a child neurologist, nurses, a clinical psychologist, a speech therapist, and members of our Developmental Psychiatry Unit team, usually a child psychiatrist and a psychiatric social worker; the latter was the same social worker who had received the referral from the child health station nurse. The Screening Clinic also accepted referrals from sources other than child health stations: from the Pediatrics Department itself, from the Speech and Hearing Clinic, from day care and other early childhood centers, and by the parents themselves. The Screening Clinic eliminated many tedious and time-consuming trips to separate hospital clinics, particularly those which had staff involved in the Screening Clinic. Through brief child-parent interviews by each specialist with three or four children, and a one-and-one-half hour conference of all Clinic staff, tentative conclusions were reached concerning the needs of the child and his family. Referrals were made to the clinics most suitable for answering these needs.

Once the developmental, including emotional, disorders of children and their families had been confirmed in the Screening Clinic, our child psychiatrist and psychiatric social worker directed them to the Developmental Psychiatry Clinic of our Developmental Psychiatry Unit. In the Development Psychiatry Clinic child and parents participated in a comprehensive evaluation of their assets and needs. The evaluation team consisted of a child psychiatrist, a clinical psychologist, a psychiatric social worker and a psychiatric nurse. Therapy was not alien to these evaluations. Each team appraisal included an evaluation conference at which conclusions were reached on the child's and family's disorders and strengths, and recommendations were made for treatment, education and still further study.

Some children whose problems were not too severe could be referred to regular community day care centers and Headstart programs; some children required the therapeutic education offered by the Therapeutic Nursery, a part of the Developmental Psychiatry Unit program; but for other children, suitable educational and therapeutic services took months to find or were unattainable. All children and families referred to us from various sources were first screened for their suitability for participation in our service. They were then followed at varying intervals through the several programs of the Developmental

Psychiatry Unit. Our functions of mental health consultation, especially to child health stations, in the Pediatric Developmental Screening Clinic and through our Developmental Psychiatry Clinic have been briefly described. In the past two years some of these functions, especially those shared with other clinics serving children, have changed to some degree; however, the purpose of the cooperative activity remains the same. The number of complete teams in our Developmental Clinic has increased to two.

Therapeutic education, the main form of treatment available to the children of the Developmental Psychiatry Unit, has been offered for the past eight years by the Unit's Therapeutic Nursery, called the Pre-School Project. This nursery was first housed outside the hospital in a community church. Lack of financial support for the nursery's housing has necessitated three additional moves; however, this nursery has succeeded in remaining in the community. It would appear that a location outside the hospital is preferred by the nursery's families. Another Therapeutic Nursery, the Pre-School Readiness Project, has been operated jointly for the past three years by the Developmental Psychiatry Unit and the Office of Special Education of the Board of Education of the City of New York. This nursery is located on the floor devoted to child psychiatry within Harlem Hospital. Therapeutic education is accomplished in both nurseries through clinical-educational teams. Teachers, psychiatric social workers, clinical psychologists and child psychiatrists maintain individual and group communication with all families; in the hospital, nurseries, at home and wherever families lead them. Both nurseries have morning and afternoon groups of six to ten children. On the average, they remain in the nursery from one to two years.

In 1970 the Unit's mental health consultation program in day care centers was expanded from work with two day care centers in any one year, to consultation with eight day care centers. This expanded work has been the result of collaboration with Sheltering Arms Children's Service, a voluntary agency, and was supported by a three-year grant from the Foundation for Child Development. Day care consultation teams—originally a psychiatric social worker and a child psychiatrist from the Developmental Psychiatry Unit—became teams of two or three mental health workers from the Harlem Unit and Sheltering Arms Children's Service. They conducted a study of one child, individual interviews with directors, teachers, family counselors, classroom observations and a child study conference in each of the eight day-care centers once every month. Child study conferences were attended by all of the teachers, counselors and directors in a center. Day care centers organized and sponsored by community groups in New York City are now largely financed through the Agency for Child Development of the Human Resources Administration. The consultation program to the eight centers just described reached the end of the three-year period of its supporting grant in December 1973. At this time, Sheltering Arms Children's Service and the Harlem Developmental Psychiatry Unit are planning continued collaboration. The consultation program is being maintained during the interim.

A few years ago, a small boy, his grandmother and his aunt arrived for a morning appointment that the grandmother had initiated with our Developmental Psychiatry Clinic team. The three-year-old's mother joined us a few minutes later. The young mother had absconded from a state mental hospital, apparently upon hearing of her little son's intended visit to our Clinic. Our small room was crowded. The clinical psychologist and I shared an interview with the small boy and his family. After a few moments during which the team consulted with one another, the psychiatric social worker conducted a brief interview of her own. She anticipated seeing the grandmother alone at another visit prior to the evaluation conference.

During and after my own participation in our lively interview, I recorded what I saw and heard in a psychiatric report. In it I described, in the words of his grandmother, three-year-old Leslie's "presenting problem," its history, the history of his growth and development, the family's history, including that of the extended family in New York and the South, my observations on Leslie's behavior during the interview, and his play with family dolls. A final section of the report, labelled Psychodynamic Summary, described for our Developmental Psychiatry Clinic team in concise terms, but in nontechnical language, my estimate of the effects of nature, nurture and trauma on Leslie's development in his family.

After the initial interview and the psychiatric social worker's second visit with Leslie's grandmother, each member of the clinic team shared his report of his contact with Leslie and his family in the evaluation conference. The team decided where to go from there; and in the subsequent chapters, we will follow the team in its work. The team, whether evaluating a child and his family, in its day-to-day contact with young children in the Therapeutic Nurseries, or in its discussions with teachers in day care centers, is concerned with the young child's development within his family from the time of his conception, and the current and past history of his family in its community and culture.

Psychodynamic givens in the study of a child's development include drives for sex and aggression. They also include rudiments of an ego which looks toward the child's ability to cope with his inner and outer world. With these drives he can achieve motor skills, gradually refine his sensory perceptions and cognitive abilities, develop language and increasingly more mature emotional responses. But first he must feed at the breast or be cuddled there while he sucks from his bottle. In this way he comes to know he is loved, is worthy of being fed. This act of trust is for all babies the cornerstone of development, making possible not only physical growth and development, but the growth of a person who can love, work, act, and make his contribution to the world. Erik Erikson (1959) made plain the commonality of this experience in his paper, "Ego Development and Historical Change," when he said,

... students of history continue to ignore the simple fact that all individuals are born by mothers; that everybody was once a child; that people and peoples begin in their nurseries; and that society consists of individuals in the process of developing from children into parents [p. 18].

In other words, young black children in Harlem have the same developmental tasks to perform as do all other children, regardless of whether their families have fathers, no fathers, or multiple mothers. They must discover how to trust, even love, at the breast. On this point, Erikson (1959) says in another essay, "Growth and Crises of the Healthy Personality," "... the baby also develops the necessary groundwork to get to be the giver, to 'identify' with her [the mother] [p. 58]." He must also separate himself from her and become his own boss. His ability to do this, to achieve his own sense of autonomy, is a reflection of the parents' dignity as individuals. The developing child needs ideal images with whom he may identify, heroes whom he may emulate.

What, then, are the main factors to consider in evaluating the press toward optimal development? The first and most elemental area is the child's "nature;" that is, his constitutional makeup, effected by genetic and congenital factors, evidence of which may be seen in his physical makeup, and even his temperament in the newborn period. An infant born in poverty in the Harlem community has a strong chance of being born prematurely, or, even if he achieves full-term birth, may be so small that the physical component of his ego is impaired. His mother may have been malnourished during her pregnancy, or ill without adequate medical care, or an addict, and her child can be born small, weak, and addicted to a habit-forming drug.

These are some of the reasons for the high incidence of minimal brain dysfunction or developmental lag, diagnoses which we currently frequently use in describing impaired "nature" in Harlem children. The diagnosis minimal brain dysfunction means to us the presence of a cerebral deficit, usually difficult to localize, and with slight, if any, recognizable motor effects. Speech delay and perceptual problems are among the developmental interferences experienced by the minimally brain injured child; although in an environment of adequate nurturing many of these children compensate for their difficulties, and achieve overall good functioning. Brain impairment, in a setting which provides inadequate nurturing, often dooms a child to developmental failure. The hazards for the combination of impaired nature and poor nurturing are extremely high in Harlem.

Another major area of concern, therefore, must be the "nurture" of the child. That is, once born, is he cared for, is he loved, is he "seen" as a person in his own right, does his daily life prove that people can be trusted, that the world is a stable and friendly place? Too often, in Harlem, conflicts arise that may interfere with the child's nurture. Has a sister been born nine months after his own birth? His need to so quickly share mother's love may arouse conflicts which interfere with his nurture. If his mother cannot buy sufficient bread for herself, or milk for him, or if his father must leave home to keep the "welfare check" coming in, his nurture will be interrupted.

"Noxia," the third major area of concern, is trauma, severe injury. It may be physical or emotional. One terrible instance of noxia, is the father who came home stoned one night and picked his 18-month-old boy out of his crib, cradled him in his arms, walked out on the fire escape and started to jump; that boy never developed speech. That event was noxious, traumatic to the black child. We lost contact with that little boy when he was three, then found him again when he was eight. He was psychotic and had to be hospitalized.

Nature, nurture, and noxia do not exist alone in Harlem. They are intertwined, interlarded, soaked through and through, and mixed up with strength, ego strength. Strength abounds in Harlem. Three hundred years of oppression and it survives. This is the task in Harlem, to see strength where it exists, to expect it to be there, right there, next to, and a part of, the nature, nurture, and noxia. Even anger may show strength. It can sustain a child and protect him until he is helped to find more suitable vehicles for his ability to love and to act.

II

NATURE

In large part as the consequence of the extraordinary achievements of medicine during the last half-century, which have virtually eradicated the killing infectious diseases and have brought greater success in the treatment of a host of other crippling and disabling disorders, brain impairment has now emerged as a major health problem ... it is to be found among the many infants who are these days born alive, only to suffer, from birth on, with irreparable brain damage. On these infants, lifelong limitations will be imposed with regard to their capacity for social adaption [Kolb, 1969, p. 4].

... since brain-injured individuals require specific types of management and education, effort should be exerted towards the development of more precise methods of diagnosis.

The concept of a continuum indicates an area within which lies the possibility of prevention of these neuropsychiatric disorders. It indicates the need for extensive studies of the factors causative to or associated with maternal and fetal factors, since these not only influence infant loss but appear to have an influence on the surviving infant. Any attempt towards preventing these neuropsychiatric conditions must of necessity be directed at the prevention of abnormal conditions associated with pregnancy and parturition [Lilienfeld & Pasamanick, 1956, p. 568].

The scene: A child health station. The entrance is the first floor to the left, reached by climbing a steep set of stairs from the street, and opening two heavy swinging doors. The "weighing room" is not crowded today, for there is a moratorium on the usual Monday well-baby conference. This is mental health consultation morning, and the two consultants from Harlem, a psychiatric nurse and myself, are part of the circle of people sitting in the middle of the weighing room. Others in the circle are Buddy, aged two and one-half, and his 23-year-old mother, Mrs. Burr; Mrs. Watson, the public health nurse, and Mrs. Brown, her assistant; Mrs. Tait, the nursing supervisor; a family assistant, and two clerks. Drs. Wolfgang and Johnson, two pediatricians, are last to join the circle. Buddy left the circle. He ran and fell about the room with abandon. His movements seemed aimless. I stooped in front of him and stopped him in his course. He struggled briefly and his small body stiffened. His eyes were fixed in a steady gaze, up and away from me, and he gave the appearance of not seeing me; but he saw me. His avoidance of eye contact was purely voluntary. Holding Buddy firmly by the hand, I picked up a small chair and led Buddy back to the circle where his mother sat tight and motionless. She did not immediately look at Buddy when I helped him into the small chair near her, and sat down next to them. I asked Mrs. Burr questions about her pregnancies (she had had two miscarriages), and the details of her pregnancy with Buddy, his labor and delivery. He was his mother's only child. To my amazement, Buddy drew a circle, played "telephone" (he had no real speech), and tapped a pencil three times in imitation of the psychiatrist. This was not behavior I would have expected of a child less than three years old. He was poorly coordinated, I found, as we played together trying to keep a balloon in the air.

While Buddy was playing with toys, I again turned my attention to Mrs. Burr. Asked to recall something of her own life story, she told of living in New York alone with her mother until she was ten. Her mother had then married and had had four babies in quick succession; and the early adolescent girl was largely responsible for the babies' care. I commented quietly, "It must have been hard to take care of your mother's four babies when you were only a girl yourself." Suddenly Mrs. Burr looked hard at me and exploded, "What's that got to do with Buddy?" Four years later, during a "follow-up" visit and after the Burrs had participated in our Therapeutic Nursery for three years, mother and psychiatrist laughed loud and long about this verbal interchange.

Mrs. Burr married at 19, giving up her course in practical nursing when it was half completed. After many attempts to get pregnant and two miscarriages, she had given birth to Buddy. Her husband, a bus dispatcher, was making good money, and she spent her days taking care of the baby, more in her mother's house than in her own. If she didn't see her mother on a given day, she telephoned.

Mrs. Burr's own concern initiated the choice of Buddy for the morning's consultation by Mrs. Watson, the nurse, and Dr. Johnson. Mrs. Burr had been on her way out of the child health station following her visit the month before our consultation on Buddy when she haltingly confided to Mrs. Watson her worry that Buddy had not showed any signs of speaking. "Don't you think that he runs awkwardly too?" she asked. Mrs. Watson told Mrs. Burr to wait while she consulted Dr. Johnson who had just examined Buddy. Dr. Johnson responded that he wasn't worried about Buddy yet, but suggested that it might be worth while to let the Harlem consultants take a look at him on their next visit.

So there we were. Dr. Johnson seemed to be restless in the pause following Mrs. Burr's tense discussion with the psychiatrist about the relationship with her mother. The pediatrician rushed into the breach and said that Buddy did seem to be a little bit awkward, but he wondered if it were not too soon to be concerned about his lack of speech. "He looks like a bright little fellow," he added. Mrs. Watson concurred, saying, "I don't really miss his speech. He always stops at the desk, smiles, and shows me something he has brought from home."

I also thought Buddy seemed like a bright, alert boy; but the history of miscarriages in the mother, speech delay in an apparently intelligent child, poor coordination, and strabismus ("cross eye"), gave me the tentative impression of "minimal brain dysfunction." It appeared that Buddy had a strong basic constitution with the exception of this relatively mild physical or organic problem. Buddy presented no obvious emotional difficulties at that time.

We felt that Buddy would respond to education geared to his needs, with a major emphasis on various kinds of communication. This kind of education was available in our Therapeutic Nursery and we anticipated choosing this facility for him should the Pediatric Screening Clinic and our Developmental Psychiatry Clinic confirm our impressions. Therapeutic education in our nursery could provide an almost one-to-one relationship with a teacher who would have a ready ear for any attempt on Buddy's part to communicate with her. She would respond to him with feeling, but not anxiety. She would help him to initiate a task, and assist him in making the move to a new one.

Our judgment at the child health station mental health conference, was confirmed by the Pediatric Developmental Screening Clinic. Here we were able to broaden considerably our view of Buddy. He and his mother were seen by a pediatric neurologist, a speech-and-hearing therapist, a pediatrician and a child psychiatrist. The Screening Clinic conference concluded that some minimal brain dysfunction might be present, and mother and son were scheduled for further evaluation in the Division of Child Psychiatry's Developmental Clinic. A few days later Miss Spanier, a clinical psychologist, and I saw Buddy, together with his mother, in this Clinic. Miss

Spanier did not determine Buddy's I.Q. in numbers at that time, but we both agreed that Buddy had good intelligence.

Our choice, in the Screening Clinic Conference, of the Developmental Psychiatry Clinic for the Burr family, rather than the Pediatric Neurology Clinic, was determined as much by our concern for Buddy's emotional development as for his organic problem; and emotional development, we know, is based largely on the family's dynamics. Buddy's development in his family, therefore, was to be central to our understanding and treatment of Buddy. In fact, any knowledge of his parents' families of origin would inform us even more on the solution of Buddy's communication problems. Nurture is inextricably bound up with nature. Buddy's physical problems were relatively mild; his mother's dynamics were more complex.

It was no accident that Mrs. Burr exploded when I asked about her pre-adolescent and adolescent role with her infant half-siblings. She had had to give up her fun in order to take care of her mother's babies; Buddy's pregnancy and birth had interfered with the renewal of her relationship with her husband when he returned home from the armed services. The baby had interrupted her vocational ambitions. Even her miscarriages became more than a woman's usual sorrow and sense of failure to her. They were a source of many fierce ambivalent feelings. Each pregnancy was a threat of being tied down by needing to care for someone else, and of becoming bereft of opportunities to pursue her own ambitions. Each, however, gave her status as a woman. She might even have more babies than mother, and so be a better woman than she. All these were primarily "dated emotions," as Sandor Rado called them, belonging, as they did, primarily to her 10- to 17-year-old time of life.

Mrs. Burr was exact in her physical care of Buddy. He was well-nourished and well-dressed. But even in the circle in the child health station weighing room, which included persons who were strangers to the Burrs, Mrs. Burr scarcely looked at Buddy. She was angry and she was preoccupied. Her preoccupation was a barrier to communication with Buddy, although his lack of speech was first a neurological problem. Buddy lacked frequent eye-to-eye, and close listening response, touch, and shared feeling contact with his mother, his main caretaker; his speech development was even further delayed than it would have been had mother-child communication been greater. Buddy also needed the approving look in his mother's eyes which would have assured him the chance of developing a good self-image, difficult under the circumstances. He was a stumbling, awkward boy, and people rarely stopped to bestow on him looks of pride and pleasure.

However, Buddy's mother was encouraged at our estimate of her son's good intelligence and was further challenged to continue to explore Buddy's needs in the Developmental Psychiatry Clinic. She still grumbled at having to repeat her own story to the psychiatric social worker, but subsequently allowed herself and Buddy to participate in more detailed evaluation without complaint.

Buddy was accepted in the Developmental Psychiatry Unit's Therapeutic Nursery. There, Buddy's teachers stooped to listen and look at him, and told him in this manner that they were aware of his worth. They taught him to freely express sadness, fear, anger, and joy. They helped him at first to put puzzles together. He knew where the pieces should go but his clumsy fat hands would not obey him. Sometimes he would be helped with this kind of activity if he would hold a pencil, or any other rod-shaped object clenched in his left hand, while he struggled to place the puzzle piece with his right. Was the rod a penis-symbol? At any rate, his good functioning with his right hand seemed to be reinforced through this maneuver. Buddy was carefully guided into social relationships with groups of his peers. By the age of three-and-one-half he could draw well, and the other children liked to listen to him read their names pasted on their cubbies, in spite of his unclear speech. Mrs. Burr came regularly to the mother's group which met just outside the nursery room with the social worker and sometimes the educational director.

The mother's meeting room was the church's small kitchen; and the children could be seen from there by peering through a hole in the wall made for the passage of food from the kitchen into the room then used for the nursery. Occasionally a child would open the door between the two rooms and run in to see his mother. Buddy rarely did this. Mrs. Burr and the other mothers talked in their group about good ways of responding to their children, most of whom had communication problems of organic or constitutional origin. This is true of the children in our Therapeutic Nurseries today. The mothers, and occasionally a father on a holiday from work, also discussed their long-time fears, anger, hopes, and desires. By the time Buddy was four, his mother had taken a job as a part-time receptionist. In those days her face began to have a relaxed and happy look.

At the age of five, Buddy was ready to leave our nursery. He spoke almost clearly unless he was under emotional pressure. It was, however, still difficult for him to engage in conversation. He continued to avoid the gaze of an adult. He was able to read and write on an early first-grade level. This achievement had occurred almost spontaneously. Buddy's strength, and his mother's strength, had been discovered through our consultative contact with them in a well-baby station. It was further supported through their experience in the Therapeutic Nursery. Mrs. Burr had become more responsive to Buddy. We regretted that we had met Buddy's father only once, when two of our team visited their home. He is a bus dispatcher, a strong, shy-looking man. Mrs. Burr blamed her husband's shyness for his lack of participation in the work with Buddy. We were not sure that Mrs. Burr did not need to have Buddy and the Developmental Unit all to herself. Mrs. Burr also blamed her husband for her unwillingness to go into individual therapy; "My husband wouldn't like it and it might spoil our marriage," she said. I had just recommended that she apply to the Columbia Psychoanalytic Clinic for treatment. This suggestion was based on Mrs. Burr's ego strengths and the feelings which to some extent still interfered with her use of her strengths.

Our Developmental Psychiatry Unit's team discussion of Mrs. Burr's possible resistance to individual treatment took an interesting turn at the time of our final evaluation conference on the Burr family. Someone on the team raised the question of whether Mrs. Burr's therapy through the parents' group and an occasional individual session with psychiatric social worker or psychiatrist were not enough for her. Was she not now more supportive of Buddy, and pleased with her part-time job? Other team members, and I was one of them, challenged our colleagues to review our own assessment of the Burr family's ego strengths. Mrs. Burr had been with us on a daily basis for close to three years. She herself had questioned if, after the many hours spent with us "in training," we were not ready to hire her to work with us. She was indeed well-known to us to be energetic, intellectually active, alert, open to new knowledge and even warm and well-related to the nursery children. She had served as a teacher substitute on several occasions. But at times her anger would interfere with otherwise good functioning, and she and Buddy would remain at home for a day or two. In spite of our usual efforts we had not plumbed the depths of her anger. Her dependent relationship with her mother had been ameliorated but not resolved. In addition, a fuller husband-wife relationship was, we felt, within the family's reach.

Such an assessment, in my opinion, should have led to thoroughgoing psychoanalytically-oriented treatment for the mother at least. With her potential for good functioning, further realized through suitable reconstructive therapy, the Burr family might have achieved even more far-reaching positive results. Having found strength in abundance in this family, residents of the Harlem community, it was our mandate to exploit it fully. Jones, Lightfoot, and Palmer, at the May 1969 meeting of the American Psychiatric Association, described the differential selection of persons for intensive psychotherapy in three predominantly-white, psychoanalytically-oriented treatment programs. They stated that the intake workers supported a point of view which stressed

> that those people who will most benefit from intensive psychotherapy are those whose ego strengths of motivation, intelligence, introspection, delay of gratification, and repudiation of action in favor of thinking are rated highly. Invariably a black person is rated as having few of the desired ego strengths and is therefore not a good candidate for anything more than the supportive therapies [Jones, Lightfoot, Palmer, Wilkerson, & Williams, 1970, p. 80].

Could we have been influenced into limiting our expectations of this strong, upwardly mobile family by the fact that the family was black, in spite of the fact that our clinical team was black as well as white?

Mimi was eight months old. Her head bobbled

on her mother's ample left shoulder. The child health station nurse was about to weigh her. When I came into Mimi's peripheral vision, her eyes focused on me with difficulty, showing the quick, lateral, involuntary movements of nystagmus. Her face was flattened on the left and her whimsical smile was crooked. She reached across her mother's shoulder and grasped the inflated balloon which I dangled at her eye level. This was again a mental health consultation by psychiatric nurse and psychiatrist at a child station in the Harlem community. The child health station staff soon gathered in the weighing room and the conference on Mimi was underway.

Mimi's mother looked depressed. She said that she had found it hard to explain her pregnancy with Mimi to her 16-year-old daughter who was an honor student in high school. "I was not a good example for my big girl," she said. "Her daddy had left us three years before I had Mimi." Even though Mimi was only eight months old, Mrs. Smith was already worried that she was slow. At her last visit to the child health station before we saw her, she had shared her concern with the nurse. The latter told her that Mimi could be seen by the team of consultants from Harlem. Mrs. Smith said that she felt relieved since she hadn't thought anything could be done about Mimi's slowness, especially while she was still so little.

We found that many of Mimi's behavioral responses were appropriate to her chronological age; others were on a much lower level. Her best responses, however, were to us indicative of her potential for good functioning. Our diagnostic impression at the end of the consultation was "minimal brain dysfunction." We told Mrs. Smith that we were glad that she had expressed her concern to the nurse, and pointed out to her some of the age-appropriate things that Mimi could do. Mrs. Smith, by bringing Mimi to us while still an infant, increased the likelihood that clinicians, educators and family could help Mimi achieve the potential she had shown during the consultation. We referred mother and infant to the Developmental Screening Clinic and then to the Developmental Psychiatry Clinic. Mimi's assets and needs were evaluated in a manner similar to our appraisal of Buddy. During the course of the evaluation we found that Mimi's big sister Linda, a talented musician, had for several months been losing ground in her high school work and was obese. We referred Linda to Adolescent Psychiatry.

Mrs. Smith and Mimi returned to the Developmental Psychiatry Clinic once every three months, and Mrs. Smith was advised on the most effective ways of communicating with Mimi. Diminished communication, interfering with learning and emotional development, we know to be the main hazard of minimal brain dysfunction in infancy and early childhood. Mrs. Smith was encouraged to pick Mimi up from her crib or playpen frequently, to talk to her, to hold her, and to allow her to move about freely on the rug. We told Mrs. Smith that since Mimi was a "good baby" who would make few demands on her, she would need to leave definite "Mimi play times" in her schedule to insure stopping her work to speak and play with Mimi. Equally important was the fact that Mrs. Smith was participating in a plan for "leading out" Mimi's strengths and those of her big girl. Being able to share in their education made Mrs. Smith a great deal happier. Her happiness was important to Mimi's development.

When Mimi was two and one-half, we invited her mother to bring her to a Therapeutic Nursery group. Mimi was a dramatic, charming, always beautifully-dressed little girl. Her residual poor coordination, together with problems of visual perception, perhaps contributed to feelings of inadequacy; but even these she covered with a beguiling coyness. During the next year and one-half, she made good use of her nursery experiences; she excelled in social skills and was very expressive of her feelings, both of which were encouraged by her teachers. When she was four and ready to enter a regular day care center, her mother was subjected to a daytime mugging on the corner of 135th Street and Lenox Avenue. Mimi was with her. Mimi, during a routine "follow-up" visit to the Developmental Psychiatry Clinic, ventilated her feelings about the mugging, just as she had learned to talk about what happened and what she felt with her nursery teacher: "He grabbed my momma's pocketbook and turned her 'round like this. My momma fell down. That man across the street looked at us and didn't do nothing. My momma was so an-ngry! I was angry too!" This ability to ventilate her feelings, to provide catharsis for them, will, we hope, stand her in good stead for other unhappy life experiences.

Mimi's mother was bright, too. She had been taking a correspondence course in political science. With encouragement, and uplifted by her new, pleasurable images of her girls, she attended evening classes in a community college and an occasional social evening.

We could not always pinpoint where nature had gone wrong. We could with Willie. He was born at Harlem Hospital and his health and illness records were available to us. We could not blame Willie's organic problems directly on his baleful Harlem environment. Willie's mother's blood type is RH negative. Willie had to be delivered by breech extraction, because the baby was in a transverse position with his right arm hanging. In addition, during the delivery, a loop of umbilical cord had become tight around his neck. The odds were against him. When delivered, his right extremities were blue, his right shoulder edematous and flaccid; he breathed only after stimulation and the birth cry was absent. These difficulties were reflected in the Apgar score, based on a perfect score of 10. It was 2 immediately after birth, and 7 five minutes later. Willie weighed 4 pounds 4 ounces. He was given an exchange transfusion. Sucking remained poor for several days.

For his first seven or eight months, Willie was a "quiet baby;" that is, he communicated very little with his caretakers and they therefore had little need to respond to him, except for feeding and diapering. However, his physical milestones, such as sitting, appearance of teeth, and walking, were within normal limits, and when he was first placed on the floor at about nine months, his mother said that he became hyperactive. Willie's mother brought him to the Developmental Psychiatry Clinic when he was four complaining that he did not talk well. He had also bitten his three-year-old cousin, which embarrassed and angered Mrs. Martin. She claimed, too, that he could play with little cars for hours, rolling them back and forth and muttering to himself. "There's something wrong with him," she complained testily. "Leah, my daughter, is only 11 months older than he and she's like a mother to him. That boy is just like his father."

Willie's mother's complaints fit the story of birth injury and possible brain damage. Willie was at first a quiet baby and later hyperactive, a usual story in minimal brain dysfunction. His language was delayed and he perseverated, that is, repeated actions uncontrollably in his play. In my office Willie made a play for me using family dolls. His speech was not entirely clear, but he did not perseverate in his story. His anger was uppermost: "The boy was beating up the sister, the mother, and the father. The boy got in his daddy's big car and drove away." Later in the Therapeutic Nursery, Willie no longer was angry with his father. He seemed to side with him against the women in his household, mother, grandmother, and sister Leah. In his drawings he placed himself beside his big father. Willie himself was represented as slightly shorter than his father. Three tiny figures in a far corner of the paper were labelled, "Momma, my grandma, and my sister." Willie's teachers sat quietly with him to help him complete a puzzle, but they also encouraged large muscle play with big blocks and aggressive play with the inflated clown. Willie compensated rapidly for his organic deficits, and showed good progress in his therapy in the Speech Clinic. Confronted with Willie's rapid improvement, Mrs. Martin agreed and said, "Well, I guess Willie isn't so bad. His cousin, my sister's boy, is the real brat." Mr. Martin, Willie's father, had left the house just before Willie came to us. The parental battle had involved "another woman." It seemed to us that Willie associated the image of "a bad father" which his mother had given him, with his own image, of "a damaged self." Mr. Martin came to the Nursery and had several fruitful talks with the social worker. He ventilated angry feelings, and found some latent strengths. Mrs. Martin participated in the mothers' group and had some individual sessions with the social worker. A reconciliation between the parents seemed to be in the offing.

Poverty and its ills are responsible for minimal brain dysfunction and developmental lag, common diagnoses in Harlem's Developmental Psychiatry Clinic. Traumatized, undernourished mothers bear small, "high-risk" babies, some prematurely born, who thrive with difficulty. After birth, they must further survive the deleterious effects of their own environments. Knoblock, Lilienfeld, Pasamanick and others, as long ago as 1953, wrote articles documenting the relationship between poor nutrition, low birth and infant weights, and depressed infant and child intelligence. They related prenatal and paranatal maternal and fetal disorders to the whole spectrum of neuropsychiatric problems, from death of the fetus or newborn baby to childhood behavior disorders. Now that we are looking for them, we are finding large numbers of black children in Harlem who show evidence of minimal brain dysfunction. Hard-to-find deficits may be noted in the motor, visuo-motor, cognitive and perceptual areas. Emotional responses may include poor body image, apparently inadequate reality testing and intellectual and emotional inhibitions. However, these same children may have overall good basic constitutions and potentially good intelligence. As has been noted, because of poor communication with the parent or other caretaker, and conflicted emotional responses, the developmental task of the child with minimal brain dysfunction is much harder than that of the child with no such deficits. These children, as young as they are, are sufficiently aware that they are not quite "right" to feel awkward, ugly, unable to attract loving glances and words from anxious, weary mothers.

The task of our team of clinical psychologists, psychiatric social workers, psychiatric nurse, educational director, teachers and psychiatrists is to search out infants and children under the age of five, living in the Harlem Hospital Community, who have developmental, including emotional, problems; to assess their disorders and those of their families; but further to assess and provide therapeutic support for their strengths and the strengths of their families. An assessment of the constitutional basis with which we work, that is, *nature,* is an integral part of each child and family study, and provides clues for remedies directed towards compensable defects. Nature is the ground through which all development is woven.

III

NURTURE

> ... to deny, in effect, that unconscious conflicts, *as well as* external stresses, contribute to symptoms, dysfunctions, and distress on the part of those who are underprivileged is to inflict still another subtle form of discrimination upon them; it is as though one were saying that, in their case, the fundamentals of psychiatry, as to psychic structure and function (including malfunction) do not apply [Bernard, 1971, p. 76].

Children are nurtured in Harlem, in spite of stressful circumstances. They are subject to the same developmental and neurotic conflicts as are more affluent children in our city. Intervention by mental health workers in the nurturing processes of Harlem children requires something more than general sympathy or even empathy, more than willingness to share our largesse. The Harlem community requires our best understanding of familial and developmental dynamics, unconscious conflicts and dated emotions, the creation of self-images and the roles and limitations of drives, ideals and goals. This knowledge is needed in the infant day care center as well as the carpeted nursery. I agree with Sandor Rado, founder and first director of the Columbia Psychoanalytic Clinic, that psychoanalysis should begin in the nursery; that is, the best we know of emotional education should begin where nurturing begins.

In our city, the proximity of large numbers of day care centers and mental health organizations, especially those related to general hospitals, provides opportunities for nurturing persons, teachers, parents, counselors, and others involved in child care, to join with those trained and experienced in the mental health disciplines for the emotional education of children of the poor. By intervening in the nurturing of children whose families have already been subjected to considerable external stress, we may gain greater knowledge of physically damaged children, bereft of proper nurturing and scarred by trauma; we may also further open our eyes to the nuances of normal development. In the annals of child and family development among the poor, study and training, as well as the creation of service modules, have a place. The goal of emotional education for all children will thereby be served. The fundamentals of psychiatry related to psychic structure, function and malfunction do apply, as Viola Bernard tells us in "The Psychiatric Care of the Underprivileged." This knowledge helps those of us who straddle both campuses, Columbia Medical Center and Harlem Hospital Center, to engage in the mutual exploitation of strengths in the Harlem community, even our own.

The scene: Hopewell Day Care Center, located in a low-income housing project, is staffed by a director, a secretary, six teachers, two parent volunteers, a cook, a cook's helper, and one male staff member, a custodian. There are about sixty children in groups of three year olds, four year olds, and five year olds.

Jared, three and one-half, was in the three-year-old group. Mrs. Best, the director, smiled at me through the ground floor glass door, unlocked it and invited me in. Mrs. Best told me that her teachers had chosen Jared for study with the consultation team because he was "running away." In a flash he would run out of his room into the hall, and if anybody happened to be going in or out of the door of the center, he would slip outside and run down the street. This understandably frightened the teacher.

My coat stored, Mrs. Best took me down the hall and excused herself while she went in to call the group teacher. Mrs. Smith, who knew that I was coming, was quickly in the hall beside me. "Jared is really doing very well. As you will see, he is a beautiful boy. Six months ago, when he first came, he was exceedingly restless and not really toilet trained. That soon straightened out, however. We are really worried now because for the past month he has been running out of our room, and even trying to run into the street when we go on walks. Mrs. Brown, the counsellor, checked with his grandmother who brings Jared most of the time, and she said that twice he has run out of the apartment into the street."

I enter the classroom and see that Jared is indeed a beautiful boy. The teacher points him out, a brown-eyed boy with a lively Afro. He is singing, seated on the floor with others in a circle. He is next to the boy with the drum. His left hand is on the head of a girl with a red dress next to him. He seems to be of average size, his movements graceful. He looks like a miniature college boy in his dark blue turtleneck sweater and brown corduroy pants. No hint of deprivation here.

Now they are at the table for snacks. "Can I have some more?" Jared asks as he scratches his left ear with his left hand. He reaches for a sandwich, saying he wants that "stuff there" (peanut butter sandwiches). He announces to no one in particular, "I got peanut butter at home too." (I make a mental note that Jared has unwittingly denied that there is a "culture of the poor." Both his turtleneck sweater and his "peanut butter at home" indicate that Jared and his family share wishes and goals with middle-class America.)

Mrs. Early is a young, lively, white social worker in a miniskirt, who has been at the day care center for about six months. She has just told me, "I have a good relationship with Jared. Perhaps I can say I'm mad about him. Every time I go into that room, he immediately sees me and smiles; then I just have to stop and smile back." While I am observing Jared, Mrs. Early does come into the room and Jared notices her immediately. Mrs. Early goes directly to a table on the opposite side of the room from Jared and pulls up a chair next to a little girl. Almost as soon as Mrs. Early is seated, Jared rises, murmurs something about the "bathroom" and leaves the table. He wends his way over to the table where Mrs. Early is seated, moves up next to her, and with his body, separates Mrs. Early from the little girl with whom she is talking. He leans towards Mrs. Early, his face close to hers, then proceeds to the bathroom. The trip takes less than two minutes. Jared returns to the table where Mrs. Early is now standing, pushes in between Mrs. Early and a girl, picks up a piece of puzzle on the table, and says "Bye" to Mrs. Early. He runs back to his own table and sits.

Two days later, six teachers, the day care center director, the center social worker, and three consultants (two social workers and a child psychiatrist) sat in the teachers' lounge for the monthly Child Study Conference. It was January, and Jared had first come to the Hopewell Day Care Center with his pretty 21-year-old mother the preceding July. The director related this information, then turned to Jared's teacher, Mrs. Smith: "Mrs. Smith, you've had Jared for the whole time that he has been here. Give us your report." Mrs. Smith spoke of the teachers' main concern, that Jared runs out of the room, and could even get out of the building if the outside door happened to be unlocked. When he first came to the nursery, he had been exceedingly restless. "There was some question of whether we could keep him," she said, "because, although his mother had stated that he was toilet trained, at first he was not."

I had encouraged Mrs. Smith when we had met briefly in the hall to remind us in the Child Study Conference of Jared's strengths, which she had shared with me. Mrs. Smith continued: "Jared seems to be very well coordinated and especially enjoys outdoor play. He swings daringly on the jungle-gym. Jared has great imagination, if he becomes interested in a task. Sometimes he asks about his drawing or clay-work, 'Is it pretty?' "

The center social worker stated that Jared's mother, Ms. Johnson, was a student at a community college and had a job in a bank. Soon after she brought Jared to the nursery, she moved out of her parents' apartment, leaving Jared with his grandparents during the week. She moved to another borough. She worked until early afternoon, picked Jared up from the nursery, and spent late afternoon and early evening hours with him in her parents' home, then went to school in the evening. The center social worker had urged Ms. Johnson to move away from home, where she had experienced considerable conflict with her parents; she had also encouraged Ms. Johnson to have a special time with Jared daily at her parents' home.

"Yes," Ms. Johnson had related to Mrs. Early one day last week when she came to get Jared. "We've had that trouble too. There were two horrible times when Jared ran out of my folks' apartment after dark. The first time I was in a panic. It was just after work and before my classes. I had been so tired and had lain down just for a short nap. Jared was watching television. I don't know what made me wake up. My folks had gone out. I didn't see or hear Jared. The television was on, and the apartment door was open. I ran down the stairs and there he was just leaving the front entrance, and without his coat. I spanked him right there."

"The second time was only a week later. This time I was sitting with Jared in front of television. I must have dozed. Again the door was open. How long he had been gone I didn't know. In the street I didn't see him. I almost don't know where I went then. I saw the man in the apartment below crossing the street carrying Jared. It was cold and he was in his pajamas."

That night Jared had curled up under the covers in his crib in the room which he shared with his teenage uncle, and told his grandmother where he had been. "Remember, Grandma," he related, "When I dropped my toy truck in the street that time? We ran across the street, but the car got my truck. You said that the car could get me. Could it, Grandma?"

Mrs. Best and many of the teachers spoke warmly of Jared. All of the teachers in Hopewell know most of the children. "He's a smart boy; he ought to do well in public school. Some of his brightly colored pictures are on the walls of the center's hall. He shows imagination, creativity, but often isn't very sure of himself. The running away has everybody worried. We're scared to take him on trips. He might bolt and run away."

The consultants from Harlem Hospital and Sheltering Arms talked about Jared together with the teachers. The chief question was, "What can we do to help Jared here in the nursery?" We discussed the meaning of the things we knew about Jared, so that we, especially his teachers, center director and social worker, could use this information to help him with his problems within the nursery. In addition, we planned that Hopewell's social worker, Mrs. Early, would share our findings and suggestions with Jared's mother.

We knew, first, that the center staff should tell Ms. Johnson what a fine, bright, gifted boy she has. His teachers and their helpers also had to constantly keep Jared's strengths in mind. Jared is valuable in his own right, we concluded, and he is constitutionally made of good stuff. He started life, thanks to the good prenatal care his mother received, and good nutritional and other health standards of his grandmother's home, with few handicaps. Just prior to his admission to Hopewell, Jared had been taken to the Pediatrics Developmental Screening Clinic by his grandmother. Her complaint was poor speech. Although delayed language development is often one of our main clues to the presence of "minimal brain dysfunction," we found nothing to support this diagnosis for Jared. We did observe, however, that the grandmother's speech often became inaudible, and that her manner of speaking seemed to operate as a denial of what she was saying. Jared's mumbling perhaps accomplished the same purpose.

Jared at three and one-half could play and work creatively. But he would often tug at the teacher's skirts and ask her over and over, "Is it pretty? Do you like it?" We had also observed Jared leaving his play so as to engage with his eyes, or actually go to meet, one of his adult friends: the teacher of the four-year-old group, the social worker, or someone he had known briefly at the hospital. He was a "charmer." Was he also a future "underachiever?" Many times I had discussed other Jareds with eighth grade teachers. "He is functioning far below his potential," we would say. "He must know that he is a bright boy and that we all like him." Remembering such discussions, we said that one of Jared's strong points is that he makes excellent contact with others; that is, he makes good object relationships. We even found ourselves "seduced" by him, in our own need to be liked by this engaging boy. Plainly too much energy (we did not say libido) is going in the direction of charming others. He should not have to work at being a charmer, and we should not need to have him exaggerate this excellent quality. He should take our "liking him" for granted, and should not have to interrupt a beautiful drawing to check on our appreciation of him. When he did check, he somehow never got back to his "creation." He needs to know more of his inherent value to us. He should better appreciate who Jared is and what he can do.

Jared had a man in his life, his grandfather. He could identify with him at this time, which was crucial to his self-image. But the two other males important to Jared, his adolescent uncle and his father, were in trouble. Young Ms. Johnson permitted Jared's father to visit occasionally. She knew that she "freezes" on hearing Jared's father's name, and said that she never had any intention of marrying him, although her father almost forced her to do so. The non-marriage was brief and she simply did not like the man. In the nursery, the custodian was the only "good man." The center had no other males.

Parenthetically, it was interesting that the parents, mainly mothers, were "up in arms" when a man teacher was suggested for the four-year-old's group. The director had had to give up the idea immediately. One mother murmured something about "a man taking little children to the bathroom." This clearly, to most of the parents, was a woman's job. At that time, the only article of men's clothing in the three year old's dress-up corner was a fireman's hat.

But what about Jared's running away? "This is dangerous." The answer came almost in choral speaking. I took the responsibility, as the child psychiatrist present, for answering. There is the possibility of "accidental" suicide in a three and one-half year old, when he needs, on a level of unawareness, to hurt himself. Just two years before, a five-year-old child in a nearby day care center, the middle of three siblings, had died in the street under the wheels of a car. An accident? He had lived his life in the streets and knew them. But the day of his death was the first anniversary of his mother's death from a self-induced abortion. I had been with this sad boy and his sisters in the nursery shortly after their mother's death, when they drew pictures of gravestones for me. A year later, Eddie, the least favored in his great-grandmother's care because of his aggressive behavior, was hit by a car. It had also been the day following his birthday.

Jared had feelings of being deserted by his mother. Originally, there was anger too, but this had been replaced by despair. "If I destroy myself," he felt, "will she come to me, feed me, love me?" Jared's mother was trying very hard to be there for Jared. She faithfully sat with Jared from four to seven each evening. Was that not enough? Almost everybody in the nursery hugged Jared and liked it. Was that not enough? Ms. Johnson had many complicated problems and worries for her 21 years. She was making a go of it, but she was tired, and perhaps very angry at her lot. Often the best that she could do was to sleep as she sat with Jared in front of the television set.

Jared's grandmother had brought him to the Development Psychiatry Clinic just before his admission to Hopewell. However, none of the Developmental Psychiatry Unit team, including Hopewell's team of consultants, had met Jared's mother, father, uncle, or grandfather. Jared had had only two visits in the Developmental Psychiatry Clinic when his grandmother announced that she was going to enroll Jared in Hopewell Day Care Center. "His mother doesn't have the time to bring him to this Clinic, and anyway there is nothing wrong with him," she explained. She was adamant and his mother did not come to see us. We heard of Jared next when Hopewell asked us to consult with them about him. The family counselor at Hopewell in the meantime had made several home visits during which she had talked with Jared's mother, grandmother, grandfather, and even his father. She had last been to the home just before the Child Study Conference. Following this conference and with the help of the supporting social worker related to our consultation team, the family counselor interpreted our findings and recommendations to Jared's mother, his grandmother and his grandfather.

Self-destructive feelings in a preschool child are a serious matter, and we would have preferred to have Jared in our Therapeutic Nursery. Since Jared's grandmother and mother had not been open to such a recommendation, we necessarily awaited other opportunities to advise therapeutic measures for Jared and others of his family. Therapeutic education is still available through the day care center's teachers, however; and what we learn in our discussions during consultation about Jared will be valuable to many other children in the teachers' care. Self-destructive behavior in young children who symbolically count themselves as being deprived of the breast is by no means unusual.

What then were some of the things that the day care center and Jared's teachers could do to help him within their own walls? First, we thought of ways that we could see Jared "for himself." We could forego the thrill of having Jared run over to lean and look up with large eyes. We could get our thrills elsewhere. Occasionally we could make the time (there were 18 children in this group) to pull up a chair next to Jared while he was making a picture. It was not enough to say, "That's a beautiful picture, Jared." He might well have responded, "Beautiful? So what? Do you see what I put into it of me, and what it means to me?" Teachers had to know to say, "That sort of looks like a tiny baby resting happy in his mother's arms." If they were wrong, he would only shout, "No! It's a fire. The house is going to burn down;" and the same purpose, that is, expression and acceptance of Jared's feelings, would be served. Or he would look knowingly at the teacher and say, "Uh-huh, she's giving him his bottle." But if he should suddenly get angry and try to tear up his picture, that would be self-destructive and should be prevented.

Although the poor tend to be socially segregated in our society, they are not as culturally isolated as we have often been led to believe. The major values of our society are shared by all (Lawrence, 1968). A twenty-four-year-old woman with four out-of-wedlock children who had been fathered by different men said, "I don't like it that my children have different fathers." The mental health team had to learn that the poor and the black are not as different from themselves as they thought from observing their overt behavior. This knowledge on the part of the team greatly influenced their interpretations, advice, decisions and their own behavior.

Psychiatrists and other members of the team avoided technical language, and translated psychodynamic principles into the simple words and drama of everyday life. They learned to function interchangeably with other members of the team because of their long-time communication with each other. Each shared the body of knowledge of his discipline with his teammates. Through the study of children and their families, our understanding of psychodynamics was constantly being enlarged.

The team continues to find new ways of functioning. In attempting to respond to families with recognition of their needs and their strengths, and in offering them assistance, members of the team often find themselves in homes, nurseries and schools, and in contact with other agencies, making on-the-spot relationships with whomever is available. The mental health worker, even the adventurous psychoanalyst, has an important role to play among the poor. He will learn much that he can apply in a larger, more general, setting. Above all, he must not despair.

IV

Noxia

> Few would doubt that what happens to young babies as they perceive the mother and other people has profound consequences, not only for the development of the all-important first relationship to another human being ... but also for the set of expectations and feelings that will dominate their orientation to the environment as a whole and toward themselves and their place in the scheme of things [Escalona, 1968, p. 47].

> ... we suggested that "the young child's hunger for his mother's love and presence is as great as his hunger for food" and that in consequence her absence inevitably generates a "powerful sense of loss and anger" [Bowlby, 1969, p. xiii].

A severe blight among young Harlem children, as perceived by those who care for them, is the trauma of separation and loss. Not infrequently, in three successive generations, we see separation from would-be "ideal images" during the first three years of life. A young black child may suffer loss of one or both parents for economic reasons, through self-destruction or "accident," through violence inflicted by others, or through drug addiction, illness and death. These parents may range in age from 12 or 13 years to 48. A previously healthy child, because of the loss of significant adults, may be interrupted in his developmental task, and suffer regression in various areas, some of which may be long-lasting or permanent. Separation and loss during childhood is always harmful, but it is more traumatic when the loss occurs at the period when the child's overwhelming need is for sustenance; later, when "initiative" develops, and the child begins to move out into the world, the loss is not quite so catastrophic.

Separation from significant adult figures is damaging to the image of the self. It interferes with identification with ideal images, those of the missing parents. It makes it unlikely that an ego so damaged will find its way to social group acceptance. Above all, there is deep anger whose original target is the lost person; but the target easily fades and the anger becomes all pervasive. It remains as years pass.

Susan, four years old, was left chiefly in the care of her grandmother. She had no father. Her mother was a fearful, dependent person who functioned best when she was working, and therefore was not threatened by the need to care for her child, although her four year old was no more than normally dependent. I visited the grandmother's neat home and was graciously served tea. When I asked the grandmother where she grew up, she responded, "In a little Georgia town. I always say that my mother gave me away to my grandmother. My mother raised my child, though."

Susan had come to our attention in a day care center. Her anger, self-destructive fantasies and literal demands to be fed brought her into therapy at our Developmental Psychiatry Clinic, but only after a year's delay due to scheduling problems. In therapy she dictated this poem, which speaks of the absent ego ideal—the mother—and the disappearance of the child's ego:

> They were walking along
> They had no mother
> They got so tiny, that
> Children couldn't see them.
> They got so tiny
> That they disappeared.
> They were never
> Back again.

In a second verse of this poem, to which she gave the title "Susan and Bobby," cries and rage found acceptance by new ego ideals, her "twin" black and white co-therapists. This acceptance promoted new ego growth:

> They cried and cried
> And cried
> They cried so loud
> That they grew
> Real Big
> They grew so tall
> That they bumped

> Their heads
> Up on the sky.

Three months after her first poem Susan dictated:

> Linda was
> A little girl
> She was walking
> Along
> She had lots
> Of sisters
> And she had
> A thousand
> Mothers,
> She had
> Two aunts
> And
> She was cute
> And
> She was happy
> And they all
> Lived together
> In a little
> Yellow house.

When separation and loss are devastating, anger is severe. The nurse had brought a 20-year-old mother, Ms. Jones, into the well-baby station for consultation with the psychiatrist. The woman was accompanied by two-year-old twins, a boy and a girl. The twins would talk to everyone in the house but the mother. The mother had been accused of "battering" her seven-year-old daughter Patsy, who had then been removed to a small state school. During the consultation, the twins rarely made physical contact with the mother. As the mother talked, Sandra, the girl twin, small and thin, began to cry. Everyone in the circle except the obese mother shifted his posture in the direction of the child. One of the conference participants said to the mother, impatiently, "Pick her up." "What do you want me to do, pet her?" retorted the mother. "That's what ruined my Patsy. My mother pet her." "You mean that your mother petted her more than she pet you," the psychiatrist proposed. "My mother didn't raise me. She sent me to my grandmother's when I was a baby." This mother had little insight into her own feelings of abandonment at this time; nor of their significance in her relations with her children.

Three generations of loss, rage at loss and destructiveness haunted this family. Ms. Jones had the support of a social service organization and had sought health care for herself at a large voluntary hospital, prior to our meeting her in the child health station conference. However, following the conference we invited Ms. Jones to the Developmental Psychiatry Clinic for further evaluation of the twins, Sandra and Sandy. We communicated by telephone with Ms. Jones's doctors at the voluntary hospital, who were pleased to know that she was getting additional help for herself in the Developmental Psychiatry Unit. Ms. Jones was pregnant when we first saw her and the twins, in the child health station. Later, after many discussions with the nursery social worker, she decided not to offer the new baby for adoption, but to keep him herself. He was a beautiful, well-developed boy, and she celebrated his birth with her family in a joyful, festive manner.

When the infant was a month old, the mother and her children were spending the night in the maternal grandmother's crowded apartment. At home, the baby had a crib; at grandmother's he slept in a bed with his mother. During the night she awoke to find that the baby had fallen between the bed and the wall. She was terrified; but he ate and slept well, and she assumed that he was all right. One week later, while she was feeding the baby at home, Sandra called out, "Mommy, Sandy is out of the window." She ran to find Sandy leaning out of the window, but safe. When she returned to the baby, he was choking. He had inhaled his milk. While she frantically waited for the police, the baby died. She had forgotten that there was an orthopedic hospital across the street.

After the baby died, Ms. Jones came to the clinic full of fear, rage and guilt. The autopsy showed that the baby had fractured his skull, probably the result of the fall from his bed at his grandmother's. Sandy showed guilt too. He had been bad and had, he felt, hurt the baby. Sandra had grown thinner. As the mother revealed her feelings, and Sandy revealed his, the mother, seated in the clinic room, suffering written on her face, at last literally opened her arms to Sandra. The twins were admitted to the Developmental Psychiatry Unit's Therapeutic Nursery; Sandra gained weight; the mother joined the Nursery's mothers' group and was seen alone each week alternately by the psychiatric social worker and the psychiatrist. Ms. Jones's own need for maternal care seemed almost insatiable. However, her desire to be an adequate mother was equally great. Herein lay some hope.

Preston, a five-year-old black boy, lost his father, his ideal image, through separation. He repeated automatically, "My father is on Long Island." His mother had been separated years before from her mother; his 15-year-old half-sister lived with this grandmother. Preston drew a stiff but excellent picture of a boy. The story of his picture read in part: "And his Daddy went to Long Island and fell out of the bus, and he stepped down and he's dead." Preston was preoccupied with the loss of a father image at a time when a father was needed on which to pattern his own male aggressive image, his own initiative. Anger at loss was the predominant feeling. Preston at the time of his story was doing well at school and was conforming in his behavior at home. Only during his therapeutic hour did he reveal his anger.

Contacts with children and their families in the Developmental Psychiatry Clinic are necessarily brief. Any one of a team of psychiatrists, psychiatric social workers, clinical psychologists, psychiatric nurses and teachers provide brief therapy, including catharsis for trauma. The team acts on demand at the clinic or nursery, in homes, day care centers, other preschool programs and in city shelters. Simulated action or massive and dramatic therapy are regularly used as rescue operations when intrapsychic and familial conflicts are urgent. Impromptu drawings, stories and play with family dolls are constantly used for catharsis of feelings. A three year old, given a handful of family dolls immediately tells the story of the fighting mother and father. "The baby is crying. She is hungry. They ain't fighting any more. The mother will get the baby some food." The child needs no other props. The story is pressing. Her feelings are accepted in all seriousness and she is coached to express herself fully.

These children's stories often sound like psychotic productions; however, unbelievable as they are, they contain a great deal of reality, and in their telling it is no longer necessary for the child to separate himself from the reality. He has an ally in the therapist. His ego can go about its integrative functions. His ally has recognized the strength of his ego and has given it validity by accepting the child's anger or badness. The ally even says, "You don't have to hurt yourself. It's all right to be angry, and scared." This is massive intervention, evacuation of feeling, freeing of the ego for integrative activity, and putting oneself on loan as an instant ideal image.

A three-year-old girl lived with her grandmother, older brother and younger sister; her mother had been killed on a roadside in the South. Mary and her grandmother had four sessions of simultaneous catharsis for their trauma, in a well-baby station and the Developmental Psychiatry Clinic. During the sessions, Mary evacuated not only her anger at the loss of her mother, but previous conflicts and anger she had felt when her sister was born. After this very brief therapy Mary was enrolled in a good day care center, where she functioned well. Every six months, up to the present—a period of six years—she has returned to the clinic for "follow-up."

James, Mary's older brother, was five at the time of their mother's death. Their grandmother found this boy pleasing because of his almost completely conforming behavior. We did not see James until he was 11. His grandmother, previously unwilling to bring him to Child Psychiatry, whispered at the beginning of James' visit when he was 11, "Maybe he is too much like a girl." He had had asthma attacks regularly for four years, and in spite of absences from school, had remained a good student. He avoided eye contact with the psychiatrist and scarcely let his voice be heard. He told the therapist that he never gets angry at anybody and that he cries, but he can't remember when. He did not cry when his mother died, nor did he cry at the funeral. He had had a dream of a Frankenstein monster, in which James grabbed a tree and ran the monster through and through.

This bright boy's dreams are indicative of the period in his ego development and his sexual development when the massive trauma and loss occurred. He had just begun to function as an aggressive, moving male. James experienced confusion in his ego identity at the time of his severe loss. Was he a bad boy? Had he himself, with his new sexual powers, aggressiveness and anger, killed his mother? If so, he felt the need to give up his sexual-aggressive actions and fantasies. He dreamt of not being able to find his home in Harlem, where he now lives, and thought that he might be living in New Jersey, where his grandfather (estranged from his grandmother) lives. He commented, "I don't like putting things together." James' dream assisted us in helping him to identify his ego ideal, his grandfather. Even his grandmother agreed that he was a good man, although they had not been able to get along with each other. James had associated the idea of living in New Jersey with his grandfather, with the dream of not being able to find his home in Harlem. For the first time he allowed himself to "put together" the things regarding his ego identity.

Our massive approach to intervention and therapy utilizes the adult worker as an ego ideal. Black anger—the patient's and occasionally the therapist's—also becomes of service to the ego in these brief therapies. The adult steps into the drama, which portrays the young developing ego doing battle with trauma and loss. The losses are those of ego ideals who not only have provided suitable patterns for imitation, but have also offered acceptance of children's developing ego images, their characters, temperaments, behavior, mental functioning and feelings. The therapist fills the part of the missing member of the cast. He, too, is accepting of these growing persons and their feelings, even anger and fear.

A three-year-old boy was brought to the clinic by his mother's boyfriend. His mother was a drug addict and had been hospitalized. Jamie had been hospitalized too, and had bitten the admitting psychiatrist. He was beautiful, broad-shouldered and "tough," which is to say I immediately admired his strength. He did look as if he would bite and, informed by intuition, I sat on the floor in front of him. He towered over me and growled, "I'll hit you with the chair, I'll burn you with fire, I'll bite you." There was a long pause; our eyes met and I responded slowly. "James, you're scared." He came into my arms crying.

There had been something good about his absent ego ideal, his mother, and her care. I stood, for the time being, in her place, openly aware of a ready, strong, positive feeling toward this boy. His anger and aggressiveness had served a protective purpose until I arrived. At a time when development of autonomy was for him the essence, his anger had been integrative in relation to hard realities. When he no longer needed his anger, he could offer his three-year-old fears to his substitute, but nonetheless real, ego ideal. This substitute did not simply bolster the developing ego; she also served the vital functions described, especially acceptance of the developing ego at a time of crisis.

In another example, Susan, our poet, whose story has been told, had co-therapists, one black and one white. It was the final session after two years of once-a-week therapy. On this occasion, the two therapists were seeing Susan successively. I was the second therapist. As I opened the door, a fecal odor greeted my nostrils. I could not hide my surprise and curiosity. The first therapist commented easily, "We closed the window; there was a bad smell outside." The first therapist retired. Susan continued to paint, apparently happily. Soiling had been one of her old symptoms, but she had never before soiled in the therapeutic hour. "Susan," I said, holding her close to me, "let's go to the bathroom. I will help you." Susan said quickly, "Nothing is the matter. I don't need to." Then watching out of the side of her eyes, "Would you really?"

This was the final test for this black therapist, rather than for Susan. Would I truly be able to accept this "worst" of Susan, her soiling? The worker's black anger, impotence, frustration and confusion, in a setting where no day turns out the way it was planned, must be noted. Forced intervention and massive use of the self wherever one finds oneself, in well-baby station, clinic, school, or on the street, for long blocks of time, in atmospheres of extreme tension, is at the very least draining of physical and emotional energies. One is reminded of how it felt riding ambulance at Harlem Hospital, 24 hours on and 24 hours off. That was in 1940. Historical perspective, both in an intrapsychic sense and in a social sense, must be achieved as one participates in the struggle on a daily basis.

V

HASSON:
A BRIEF MULTI-AGENCY STUDY

> Those individuals who are at once both socially deprived and in psychiatric need are burdened by composite problems, and composite problems require composite remedies [Bernard, 1971, p. 62].

> All children are reticent. They see the bare bones of experience, and they are absolutely accurate in their fantasies [O'Gorman, 1972, p. 18].

All children have mothers and are born into families, but not all are so burdened by the composite problems, the terrible bare bones of experience of the McManus family. In the words of our time, this is a multiproblem family requiring a multiagency approach. Our child health station consultants saw the beauty and strength of the black-American mother and her three children with African names. These qualities, as well as the multiple problems that threatened to swallow this family, demanded multiple identification on the part of our interdisciplinary team; identification with each other, with this family and with the five or six agencies with which the family had contact. All of us had to achieve multiple and mutual responsibility.

Mrs. McManus did indeed look flat, and yes, surly. She was a tall, black, should-have-been handsome woman, who had walked in with a limp. She had three children with her: Hasson, aged four, Sadgia, three, and Kahjia, two. Our curiosity did not permit us to wait long before asking the source of her childrens' names. She told us with real pride that Hasson meant "warrior," Sadgia, "beautiful," and Kahjia, "princess." "These are African names."

We were having an interdisciplinary, interagency consultation on the McManus family at the Mt. Morris Child Health Station. Those present were three nurses and a doctor—Mrs. Clawson, Mrs. Gadsby, Mrs. Hampton and Dr. Leola Pride—from the child health station; Mrs. Boston, a social worker, from the Welfare Department; and Mrs. Beth Armstrong, psychiatric nurse, and I from the Developmental Unit of the Division of Child Psychiatry, Harlem Hospital Center. Mrs. Armstrong and I were the regular Developmental Psychiatry Unit Child Health Station consultation team, and it was our bimonthly consultation with the Mt. Morris Child Health Station.

It was indeed an awesome group that joined Mrs. McManus in the empty baby-weighing room in January, 1971. But Mrs. McManus had met groups of public servants of various sizes before. Two of her chief helping agencies were not even represented: the Dominican Sisters, housed in her neighborhood, and the Storefront Nursery, conducted by the poet Ned O'Gorman. It is he who freely accepts all "rejects" from other early childhood centers in the Harlem community. Ned O'Gorman has published his own volume on Hasson and his other "wild" children, *The Wilderness and the Laurel Tree.* For the purposes of this story it is important to know that Ned had given Mrs. McManus a job teaching in his storefront the previous August. Her home had been described as "utterly disheveled" by one observer, although another visitor had described it as "clean" and "light." Her children were said to be unresponsive. They babbled and grabbed food; although Ned himself said that Hasson, Sadgia and Kahjia were the "owners of beautiful myths."

We did not improve our knowledge of the McManus family a great deal during this consultation except to learn that things had been looking up for all of them since the Dominican Sisters had brought Mrs. McManus and her three children to the Storefront the previous August. The week prior to the consultation, Mrs. McManus had confided to the health station nurse, Mrs. Hampton, some very specific complaints about Hasson. She wondered if he were speaking well enough for his age, and she thought that maybe he got a little too angry when things frustrated him. The nurse had offered to have the McManus family come in when the "people from the Harlem Developmental Psychiatry Unit" would make their regular visit. Mrs. McManus also agreed to let her "caseworker" from the Welfare Department join the meeting.

Mrs. McManus was 28 years old and had four children older than Hasson living with her mother and father in North Carolina. They were all boys, and all had less exotic names than those of the younger children. Mr. McManus had been sent to prison when Mrs. McManus was four months pregnant with Hasson. Since then, Mr. McManus has been out on parole and at home several times for periods as long as six months, only to return to prison. The family visits him regularly.

Mrs. McManus's pregnancy with Hasson had been fine like all of her pregnancies. Labor had lasted for one hour. His birth weight was seven pounds fourteen ounces. Mrs. McManus had wanted to breastfeed Hasson, but did so for only one day. "I got lumps and bumps and they wrapped me. It stopped my milk." She added that she had been stopped from breastfeeding Sadgia when the child became sick, but that she had insisted on breastfeeding Kahjia the whole time; that is, until she was walking. Hasson had been close to two when she went to Flower-Fifth Avenue Hospital to give birth to Sadgia. She had left Hasson with a good friend. He had searched the house for his mother, sat and stared and began rocking. When Mrs. McManus came home with the baby, her husband was released from prison simultaneously. Hasson did not rock while his father was at home, but sat on his knee. He would throw things at the baby. His father returned to prison when Hasson was two and one-half. Hasson rocked again.

It appeared now that the environment of the McManus family had come under reasonable control.

The Developmental Psychiatry Unit, feeling from their observations of these handsome, now alert and well-nourished children that they were physically intact, suggested that the family visit the Developmental Unit evaluation team for further exploration into the emotional development, needs and relationships in the McManus family. Mrs. McManus again expressed her concern about Hasson, and said that she would ask Ned for time off and would bring all three children. The Harlem team promised to maintain contact with the other agency representatives, including the Dominican Sisters. Ned O'Gorman would see to it that we had conversation with him.

Some days later, all four of the McManus family crowded into my small office with Miss Spanier (the clinical psychologist) and me. Mrs. McManus said that she really did not think that Hasson was slow, but that she wanted to know for sure. Up until recently, she said, he had pointed to things and screamed. "Now he is saying a few words," she added. She recalled that once during her pregnancy with Sadgia, she was sitting on the side of the bed crying. Hasson had come up to her knee and very plainly said, "I love you, Mommy." There were other times during that same pregnancy when she and Hasson were very happy together. They would go to the park and have picnics. Even when Hasson was an infant and her husband was extradited to North Carolina, she felt especially close to Hasson; "I guess," she mused, "because I was so lonely." She informed us that Hasson still would not share toys with the little girls. He seemed to have no fears and recently he has been happy with a puppy which he found.

Mrs. McManus has a 29-year-old brother, and a 28-year-old sister who is less than a year older than she. She felt particularly close to another brother, Sammie, who was less than a year younger than she; in their school years she was like a mother to him. It is he who reminds her of Hasson. "Sammie was so nice." A second sister was the youngest child in the family. Mrs. McManus grew up with both parents, but felt closer to her father. He had died of a heart attack the previous March. "He had a zest for life," she said. Mrs. McManus had had her first baby when she was 15. Remaining home, she went back to school and stayed there until she was in the 11th grade. She had done well in school and wanted to be a nurse. She had left school in the 11th grade, pregnant with her second child. She had married the father of her children, over the objections of her father who thought her husband "no good," and had moved to a place in the same town, still supported by her parents. When she was 20 and had four children, she left them with her mother and followed her husband to New York. "He had gotten into trouble."

My summary was brief: The McManus family in New York seems to have survived in spite of remarkable troubles. One suspects that maternal strength is responsible.

Although Hasson had four older brothers, he is almost a "first child" in his relationship with his mother. In spite of the fact that the mother seems to depend on Hasson when she feels bereft, the child cannot be said to have a symbiotic relationship with her. He functions independently of her in his relations with others, and is in good contact with his environment. He is highly competitive with the sister next to him, but sometimes agrees to take care of the baby sister, which pleases his mother. He often represses anger in the service of maintaining his relationship with his mother.

During the evaluation Hasson did indeed scream when frustrated, particularly when his three-year-old sister took toys from him. On those occasions his mother would "help" him. Hasson hid behind his mother. He was carrying a toy gun and would smile and "shoot" it at me when resisting play with me. It seemed clear that it was Hasson's role to express much of his mother's aggressiveness, even through his name of "warrior." However, her ambivalence about her own aggressiveness perhaps showed in Hasson's inhibitions in behavior, and even in his speech. In the family interview he spoke a number of single words in response to my communications, but rarely a three- or four-word sentence.

With Miss Spanier, he was awkward in catching a ball, but otherwise seemed well coordinated. He may have had little experience in catching balls. He was responsive to the psychologist, but did not seek attention. His vocabulary approached that of a three year old. Generally, he tried to please Miss Spanier when she offered him a few tests, and showed himself to be of good intelligence. Other than "shooting" his gun with a smile, he resisted the expression of anger to anyone outside of his family circle. Mrs. McManus and the evaluators spoke of her strength that had made survival possible against great odds, and we said that her three children were in remarkably good shape. We encouraged her in her teaching at the Storefront. We also helped her to have insight into Hasson's role in her life, in the midst of her trials, and gave her evidence that she need not depend on him. Although Hasson is very conforming to adult demands, inhibited in the expression of his wishes and temperamentally less outgoing than his charming younger sister, he need not have his mother protect him. We reminded her of the similar relationship she had had with Sammie, her slightly younger brother; and again used her teaching as evidence that she need not have others thoroughly dependent on her in order to prove herself a good woman.

Mrs. McManus telephoned a year later, in June, 1972, and reached Mrs. Ricigliano, the Developmental Psychiatry Unit's coordinating psychiatric social worker. Mrs. McManus said that Hasson needed to see Dr. Lawrence, and that the Dominican Sisters had agreed with her that this was true. In dress and general appearance, Mrs. McManus and Hasson looked exceedingly well. Hasson was slender, average to tall in height and good looking. His mother was more slender than before, and tall and handsome in her Afro haircut. The last was new. But Mrs. McManus's eyes looked like those of a wounded animal. When, again in my small office, Miss Spanier asked Hasson to join her at a low table, I motioned to Mrs. McManus to sit with me in a corner opposite Hasson.

There had been more trouble, Mrs. McManus said. Her husband had been transferred from Danbury to Clinton, and had come home for a two-month stay. He had gotten into drugs during that period and had returned to Clinton. "Hasson doesn't want to talk about his father. He says that he does not miss him." However, three weeks before her visit with me they had all gone to visit Mr. McManus. Hasson had sat happily on the table and talked to his father.

Suddenly Mrs. McManus burst out, "That isn't it." Mrs. McManus then recalled for us the events of Easter Day. "I took Hasson and his two little sisters to see my brother Sammie. The children were all dressed up so pretty. I thought it was funny that I couldn't get into my brother's apartment because I had told him I was coming and he had said that he would be there all day, Easter Day. The 'super' of the building said that he thought he was there too, and he came up with the key. When the super opened the door we walked in, the children and me. Sammie was lying on the floor in a pool of blood with his throat and his stomach slashed. We all saw him at once. I screamed. Hasson just stood there and the girls were holding my knees. Hasson said, 'He's dead, Mommy. Let's go to the movies.' Sometimes I sit and dream that it was not Sammie but somebody else. I'm afraid to be in the house alone. Do you think I'm afraid that the same thing will happen to me? I didn't do enough for Sammie. He was just a year younger, but he always depended on me. If he had been with me, it wouldn't have happened. He was separated from his wife and three children down South and he was very lonely."

Suddenly I looked at Hasson. He was looking at his mother. I excused myself from Mrs. McManus and went to Hasson, asking Miss Spanier if I might speak to him. I sat close to Hasson. "You must have been very scared and sad to see your uncle dead," I said quietly. "It was a bad thing. He wasn't breathing. He wasn't smiling. He wasn't moving and there was all that blood. It wasn't even your uncle any more. He was dead and that was his body left, and your mommy had the undertaker clean his body up and take it to North Carolina and bury it in the ground. But Hasson, you still have your uncle's love, because he loved you very much."

Hasson ran from the table to the door, and stooping, I caught him in my arms. "No, no!" he cried. "I was *not* scared. I was *not* sad." I confronted him again. "It's all right to be scared. It's all right to be sad. He loved you and you still have his love. And you love him very much, and you love your daddy very much, even when you are angry that he is not with you. And you didn't do anything bad. You are a strong boy, Hasson, and your Mommy and the teachers, and Sister, and Ned, and all of us will help you. It is all right to be strong, strong like the strong things about your uncle and your daddy." We talked about his Mommy screaming and how this must have made him feel even more scared, that she was feeling so sad and scared.

It was a long few minutes, and Hasson and I were struggling physically most of that time. My impression later, however, was that I did not really have to put forth very much effort in order to contain him.

The catharsis of feeling that he experienced, I sensed, was with his consent. He became quiet and even resumed testing with Miss Spanier. I returned to Mrs. McManus. I believe that she had participated fully in Hasson's catharsis. Her eyes seemed to say so. She said that she felt very much alone and that she was glad to be a teacher-aide, that she depended on this. She recalled that her brother had come to see her on his birthday. She made him a cake and they had gone for a walk together. They were very close. I emphasized how much she had helped her brother, and now how important it is for her to continue to do things for herself in order that she can sustain herself and her children, and also help her husband as much as possible. I said that it helped both Hasson and her, and even the little girls, to be able to express their grief about her brother. I suggested that she talk with Hasson and the little girls, for a time, about missing Uncle Sammie. I offered her another appointment in a week, just to see how things were going. I asked her about her sleeping and appetite, and she said that she thought she was going to make it.

Mrs. McManus did come in a week later. Hasson was sporting a Band-aid over his left eye. Mrs. McManus said that she did not really know how he had gotten his small injury, but said that she wondered sometimes if Hasson defends himself enough with the other boys. Mrs. McManus was jubilant. She was being sent with her three children to an early childhood education meeting in London. My excitement knew no bounds. We spent our time, however, clearing out some of the remaining feelings of grief and guilt about Sammie. This was our going away present to Mrs. McManus. In the meantime, Hasson, with Miss Spanier, had performed very well on his tests, and had even begun to read. As he left, he called out quite clearly, "Goodbye, Dr. Lawrence."

What was the investment of the Harlem Hospital Center Developmental Psychiatry Unit in the McManus family? A psychiatric nurse, Mrs. Beth Armstrong, a psychiatric social worker, Mrs. Frances Ricigliano, a clinical psychologist, Miss Irene Spanier, and a child psychiatrist, Margaret Lawrence, had made a visit in consultation with child health station staff and others, had met the McManus family on three occasions on the sixth floor of the "K" building of Harlem Hospital, had visited the Storefront on the way to the Therapeutic Nursery, and had made a number of telephone calls to Ned O'Gorman, to the Dominican Sisters, to the Welfare Department caseworker and to the nurses at the child health station. A full record of these transactions may be found on Hasson's chart at Harlem Hospital. This material is in the same binder as the story of Hasson's pediatric contacts with the hospital. While there were such contacts during the period under discussion, no cross-fertilization between the pediatrics and the child psychiatry departments occurred. Such an interchange may well have been instructive as an occasion for consultation to the Comprehensive Pediatrics Clinic, or in conjunction with the regular operation of the Pediatrics Developmental Screening Clinic in which the Developmental Psychiatry Unit regularly participated.

A family visit, in this instance, would at least have cleared the air with regard to the opposing opinions of observers from two different agencies that Mrs. McManus kept a home that was "utterly disheveled," or "clean" and "light." However, Mrs. McManus had had many observers in her home; and besides, she was willing to bring the whole family to us. Additional information on this point had been revealed in the course of the year. Mrs. McManus's home had been utterly disheveled when she was in the hospital for a month because of a broken foot. A homemaker had cared for her home and children during the day, and brother Sammie at night. When she returned from the hospital, her home became clean and light. A family visit from our team, however, would have gone further than observations for cleanliness; it would have given us even greater insight into intrafamilial relationships.
    The McManus family was able to make use of the full extent of our combined skills which were based on our appreciation for its history, in two communities, North Carolina and Harlem, or perhaps four, including the two prison communities. The concern and knowledge which began with the McManus family in four primarily black communities can now extend to other families and communities. These need not be black, nor even poor. Mrs. McManus had used the nursing skills of the nurses in the child health station. Mrs. Armstrong, our psychiatric nurse, had made plain to our Harlem team the important role the nurses had played. She said that the child health station nurses picked up the cues, both that something was very wrong, and that something was right

with the McManus family, and had encouraged the mother to use the Harlem team. "Nurses are good observers," she said. "They put the notes on the blue sheets of the patient's chart which doctors forget to read. The nurse represents the whole person, mind and body of people who are not well. She gets the feeling of people who are not well on the wards, where the nurse must remain eight hours a day. If she's a good nurse, she uses herself in a 'caring' way, and knows the importance of accepting the feelings of both patients and their families. She often is the only one to be aware of entire families, and their importance to the patient." Mrs. Armstrong also served as the knowledgeable connection between the child health station, Pediatrics and Child Psychiatry, and could translate medical customs and language for Mrs. McManus. I enlarge on Mrs. Armstrong's contributions, because they are perhaps less well known than those of the rest of the team. Exchange of roles by various team members, or inclusion in the teamwork of local "self-help teams" or "talent-corps," requires, in each instance, the steady support of the discipline which brings to the team the required knowledge gained from years of training and experience in a given field.

In addition to the collaboration of the full Developmental Psychiatry Unit team, which greatly enhances individual skills in work with the family, the two-person teams are of great value. They provide consultation to the child health station, such as that offered by the psychiatric nurse and the child psychiatrist; and are used in diagnostic evaluation at Harlem. Miss Irene Spanier, clinical psychologist, and I have for a long time worked in this manner at Harlem and under other auspices. We have called our work a "screening procedure," which permits us to choose test items and parts of other clinical examinations from pediatric, neurological and psychological perspectives, choices made necessary by the historical context in which the family comes to us. It is a procedure which demands continuous contact with the "level of unawareness" of the team and of the family; it permits two not-unrelated tasks, a psychological and a psychiatric examination, to be accomplished simultaneously, with mutual interruptions possible and welcomed. These two evaluative sessions with the McManus family were "brief," even "massive-dose," family therapy.

In the three sessions on Harlem's "6K," catharsis of feeling, use of interpretation and encouragement of insight played major roles. Mrs. McManus is a capable woman, with great ego strength. In the midst of much necessary activity, she regularly practices introspection. She and her children make good object relationships, and are in remarkably good contact with their own feelings. These are their strengths, these and more. The method of providing catharsis for feeling in anticipation of potentially traumatic happenings, or after they have occurred, is an instrument which I have learned to use in many settings, whether in a middle-class home, during consultation in a day care center, or in a therapeutic nursery. It is of particular value for the preschool child. Providing for expression and acceptance of deep feeling, particularly in overwhelming situations, when denial would seem to be the only available defense, and the ego needs a temporary adjunct, may be an acute therapeutic need at any age. Given these as appropriate therapeutic and evaluative methods at any class level, given the basic soundness of the various psychodynamic, pediatric, sociological and other principles involved, I believe that these methods were applicable to the McManus family. Viola Bernard greatly informs my understanding of this and other Harlem families when she writes in *Psychiatric Care of the Underprivileged:*

> Treatability, it would appear, is a function not only of class or racial characteristics, but also of the motivation and the capacity of therapists to modify their own personal attitudes, as well as their techniques [1971, p. 77].

VI

PEDRO:
A HARLEM CHILD STUDY

Pedro was presented in seminar at the 75th anniversary celebration of the New York State Psychiatric Institute and Hospital in November 1971. During the previous summer, after three years in our Developmental Psychiatry Unit, especially its Therapeutic Nursery, Pedro had been referred to the residential Children's Service of the Psychiatric Institute. The time seemed ripe to consolidate the gains which Pedro had made at Harlem. In the residential setting we knew that he would have a stable environment, as well as the necessary therapies and education suitable to his needs. We anticipated a one- or two-year stay. Pedro's sister Maria had joined Pedro in our Therapeutic Nursery and would remain with us. His mother, in Pedro's absence, could better pursue her own educational and vocational goals. His father would become more responsive to the approaches of Psychiatric Institute workers than he had been to us, and more accessible to Pedro.

This report was prepared and written by the Developmental Psychiatry Unit Team: Frances G. Ricigliano, A.C.S.W.; Helen R. Drew, B.S.; Irene J. Spanier, M.S.; Margaret Morgan Lawrence, M.D.; and Katrina de Hirsch, F.C.S.T.

In the chapter that follows, individuals on the Developmental Psychiatry Unit team at Harlem report their work with Pedro and his family, and their findings. Mrs. Katrina de Hirsch, consultant in language pathology at Psychiatric Institute, shares her study of Pedro and its interpretation which followed his referral for residential education and treatment.

Pedro was born on July 17, 1966 and as this clinical session begins he is five years and four months old. In 1964 Pedro's father left Santo Domingo and settled in the Harlem Hospital Center community. His mother followed a year later. Pedro had a sister, Maria, shortly before he was two years old. In January 1969, when Pedro was two and one-half, his mother brought him to the Pediatric Clinic complaining that Pedro had a cold. She took this occasion to tell the doctor that Pedro was so active that he tired her, although he was not a destructive child. The doctor noted her complaint and then added that the little boy was active, alert and playful. Except for a mild upper respiratory infection, he found Pedro normal.

Pedro's mother had also complained of what she assumed to be Pedro's hyperactive behavior to the Central Harlem Child Health Station nurse-in-charge. She had been faithful in bringing her son to the child health station. The nurse suggested that she could have Pedro seen by a child psychiatrist from Harlem, who might help the nurses and doctors at the health station to decide if Pedro and his family required any help. The nurse referred to the possibility that the child health station might refer Pedro to the psychiatric nurse/child-psychiatrist team from the Developmental Unit in Harlem's Division of Child Psychiatry. Although the pediatrician, nurses and consultation team conferring at the child health station agreed that the two-and-one-half-year-old Pedro appeared to be a bright and alert boy, his mother's description of Pedro's constant running about the house that kept her fatigued, and her additional concern that he seemed slow to speak, made staff and consultants agree to refer Pedro to the Pediatric Developmental Screening Clinic at Harlem. The following Monday, Pedro was one of four preschool children examined in the Screening Clinic by a pediatrician, a pediatric neurologist, a speech diagnostician and a psychiatrist. A nurse in the Screening Clinic helped Mrs. M. to fill out a form giving Pedro's developmental history and outlining his mother's complaints and concerns.

Presenting Problem

In the Screening Clinic, Mrs. M. enlarged her concerns about Pedro. She was worried that he was not speaking. He did not "pay attention." He seemed to be afraid of swallowing, and sometimes gagged.

Pedro had said "Mama" and "Dada" at one year; he had said little else between the ages of one year and two and one-half. His motor development, however, seemed normal, and by the age of one he "ran wild" in the street. Mrs. M. admitted to being "nervous, tense and irritable" during this period; and since Pedro would seldom do what he was told, his mother frequently found herself hitting him. On the other hand, after he started walking he played alone a good deal. When he was with his mother, however, she felt unable to hold his attention.

During the first six months of his life, Pedro would take as long as an hour to finish six ounces of milk. He was given solid food at two months, and soon after he bagan to hold his food in his mouth and then spit it out. During his second year, when his mother would force him to eat baby food, soup, or spaghetti, he gagged and seemed afraid to swallow. Later he seemed to want to feed himself, but Mrs. M. felt that this would be too messy.

DEVELOPMENTAL HISTORY

Mrs. M. gave the following history of her pregnancy with Pedro: there was slight vaginal bleeding between the first and third months. During her third month, she had fallen on the stairs with no apparent injuries; and again, in her eighth month, she fell in the street on her abdomen. Pedro was born in Metropolitan Hospital weighing nine pounds. On examination he was described as a normal infant.

All developmental milestones were within normal limits. He walked at nine months, and could toilet himself at two years three months. His weight and height remained between the 80th and 90th percentile.

Personal History

When Pedro was two months old, Mrs. M. went to work at a factory for eight hours a day. She left Pedro with the building superintendent. This caretaker would prop Pedro on the couch in front of the television set and leave him alone. When Pedro began to walk, Mrs. M., on returning from work, would sometimes find him alone outside the super's basement apartment. Pedro stayed with various babysitters from his second to his 18th month. Mrs. M. rarely talked to Pedro; she was having a great deal of trouble with her husband, and felt depressed most of the time. When Mr. M. finally left the home in January, 1969, Mrs. M. took Pedro into bed with her, although the children had a bed of their own. She said that Pedro was scared, but admitted that she was frightened too.

Family History

This history is a composite of the history obtained by the Pediatric Developmental Screening Clinic, and the family history as elicited later by the Developmental Unit of the Division of Child Psychiatry.

Mrs. M. was born in Santo Domingo, Dominican Republic, and was her mother's only child. She and her mother lived primarily with her maternal grandmother. Her father lived with another woman, and had children by her. When Mrs. M. was 12 years old, her mother died after a long illness, and her grandmother assumed full responsibility for her. Mrs. M.

believed she had heard her mother calling to her both the night before and the night after her death. Her grandmother was strict and very religious, and although Mrs. M. was highly emotional in her own religious activities, she rebelled against her grandmother's strictness. Her relationship with her father was strained, but she saw him frequently. She felt that he cared little for her and had cared little for her mother.

Mrs. M. went to college in Santo Domingo for about a year, and there met her husband. His brother was the editor of a student publication to which she submitted poems and stories. They married in 1964. Shortly afterwards, Mr. M. left for New York City and his wife joined him in late 1965. In the United States, Mr. M. worked as a laborer and Mrs. M. had infrequent employment. She began work in a factory two months after Pedro was born. The M.'s had serious marital problems and separated in January, 1969. Just before their separation, Mrs. M.'s grandmother died. Mrs. M. developed many complaints, including headaches, heart palpitations, insomnia and weakness. Shortly after bringing Pedro to the Pediatric Developmental Screening Clinic, Mrs. M. sought help for herself in the adult psychiatric clinic. The diagnosis of "anxiety reaction" was made. She began therapy at Harlem and then continued later at the Bronx Mental Health Center. The change was made in order that she might have a Spanish-speaking psychiatrist.

Following Pedro's entrance into the Therapeutic Nursery program in the summer of 1969, Mrs. M.

had numerous contacts with various members of the Developmental Psychiatry Unit's interdisciplinary team. With her deep dependency needs, she required constant support, reassurance and direction, all of which were made possible within the context of a team approach. During Pedro's first summer in the program, Mrs. M.'s anxiety and depression, probably in response to the death of her grandmother and separation from her husband, were so overwhelming that she threatened suicide. At this time she avoided her male psychiatrist and told Pedro's teacher of her self-destructive feelings. Ventilation with this teacher and a female child psychiatrist in the Unit team resulted in prompt relief from her anxiety and depression. Subsequently, Mrs. M.'s feelings so immobilized her from time to time that her daily functioning and Pedro's attendance at the nursery suffered greatly. While demanding constant support, she maintained considerable distance from members of the Unit team by pleading language difficulty when, in fact, she spoke and understood English quite well. At the same time, she often sought a familiar relationship with team members, asking personal questions and inviting them to her home.

Mrs. M. was strongly attached to her children, and from their infancy sought for them the help they needed. Preoccupation with her own feelings, however, consistently interfered with her communication with both children. She felt alone and isolated except when she was romantically involved; and in neither case was she emotionally available to the children in a stable, nurturing manner. She worried about Pedro's difficulties, but was not able to alter her relationship with him significantly in order to better meet his needs. She was saddened and dejected when the recommendation was made that Pedro receive inpatient help. However, she appeared to be able to accept the referral, primarily because of her intense dependence upon the staff and their constant support. Mrs. M. was able to maintain her contact with the Therapeutic Nursery even after Pedro was no longer attending because his sister Maria was still enrolled there. Mrs. M.'s questions about the referral to Psychiatric Institute, however, indicated her projection of hostility, guilt and separation anxiety. She, however, began to work part-time; Maria was then cared for after school by a warm babysitter. With this arrangement, the family seemed to achieve a tenuous stability.

SUMMARY OF NEUROLOGICAL FINDINGS

The pediatrician on the Pediatric Developmental Screening team confirmed the findings of the doctor in the Pediatric Clinic: all systems appeared to be normal.

Neurological examination of both Pedro and Maria revealed light brown *café au lait* spots, which proved to have no pathological significance. Vision, gait and reflexes were normal. Pedro's skull X-ray revealed no bony abnormalities or intercranial calcifications. The sella turica outlines were normal. There was no evidence of intracranial pressure.

Although minimal brain damage was raised as a possible diagnosis, neurological examination offered no positive confirmation. Referral to the Developmental Unit of the Division of Child Psychiatry was made chiefly because of the evidence of the M.'s intrafamilial conflicts and Pedro's developmental conflicts. Although Pedro's hyperactivity and language delay were not significant at two years seven months, family and developmental history indicated remedial measures. Gagging, which was earlier noted in the mother's statement of Pedro's "presenting problems," was at no time observed while Pedro was under our care.

Summary Report from the Therapeutic Nursery

Pedro came to the nursery early in June, 1969, just prior to his third birthday. At that time the Therapeutic Nursery was on the ground floor of a church rectory. Pedro shuffled into the nursery room, followed by his mother. She was pushing Pedro's sister, Maria, in her stroller. Pedro flitted about the room, observing its contents and stopping every now and then to open and shut the doors and drawers of the cupboards, the piano and the room. His skillful manipulation of these objects was startling for a child his age. He was short and stockily built; and his large, round eyes never seemed to see the adults present, or another child who arrived later. This boy approached Pedro and unsuccessfully attempted to engage him in play. Pedro had a fixed, broad smile.

However, he seemed to be aware of things going on about him without observing them directly, and with sideward glance and tilted head appeared to be listening.

During July and August, 1969, Pedro had individual play time with his teacher twice weekly for an hour. The nursery planned to move to a new location, and during the summer of 1969 it temporarily occupied a room in a public school. This room had a view of the busy intersection of 135th Street and Fifth Avenue. Pedro would say "car" while looking out of the window, and became very excited each time he saw a white automobile. His father had a white car. Pedro also shouted "Papi" or "Daddy" as he watched men passing on the street. Soon he began to say "Hi" and "Bye-bye" to familiar people. He usually played with cars by himself, but would join the teacher in play for short periods of time, and he would also count in rote fashion in Spanish from one to five.

There was an interval of about two weeks between the Therapeutic Nursery's summer and fall sessions. During that time, Pedro had an accident in the reception area of the Child Psychiatry Clinic. His mother, as was her custom, had left Pedro in the waiting room in the general care of the nurse and secretaries there, while she went to the adult Psychiatry Clinic. Pedro had already developed a close friendship with a male psychologist whose office opened into the waiting area. Often he would run into the office, pulling out the desk drawers and looking for familiar objects such as a car, a top, or a pencil.

At times he would put a chair next to the psychologist's, as if he were sitting at his desk. He could put paper into the electric typewriter, and type using two hands. He had considerable nonverbal communication with this psychologist, smiling his shy smile and waving goodbye.

On the day of the accident, Mrs. M. was in the midst of an acute marital crisis. Having quickly deposited Pedro in the childrens' waiting area, she left, with baby Maria in her arms, for her appointment. With one push of the large heavy wooden door to the psychologist's office, Pedro mashed his finger in the doorway. He did not cry. A secretary and a nurse rushed to help, but Pedro remained stiff and uncomplaining. When his psychologist friend came in sight, Pedro threw himself to the floor. The man gathered Pedro in his arms, comforted him and told him that his hand must hurt very badly. Pedro began to cry with tears and loud wails. His hand was badly hurt and bleeding; the teacher, who soon arrived, and the psychologist washed his hand and continued to comfort him. They took Pedro to the Emergency Room, continually speaking to him of his pain, his fear and his anger. As they waited in the Emergency Room, Pedro nestled in his teacher's arms. It was the first time that he had allowed this kind of direct contact with his teacher.

When Mrs. M. came in sight, Pedro quickly sat up straight and began to manipulate gadgets nearby. The teacher became a mediator between Pedro's mother and Pedro, helping her to offer comfort and sympathy. This was the first of Pedro's many self-destructive episodes in the nursery. They spoke of his anger toward a mother preoccupied with her own troubles and an infant sister who could be closer to mother than he. Both Mr. and Mrs. M. also seemed to be involved frequently in self-destructive acts. Pedro was often absent from the nursery. These absences were related to Mrs. M.'s emotional state. After he had been away, Pedro regressed in spoken language and in his relationships with others. A family trip to the Dominican Republic, followed by Pedro's hospitalization for a leg infection, resulted in further withdrawal and regression.

By the spring of 1970, however, Pedro's English-speaking vocabulary had increased to forty words, plus an additional five proper nouns. He had about eight short phrases, such as "Oh, how pretty"; "I don't want to"; "He's sleeping." He was able to concentrate on a single activity for longer periods, and he could even relax on his pad for ten minutes at a time. If his teacher read to him alone, he could listen to stories. He loved the out-of-doors, and enjoyed the see-saw, the sliding board and the swinging horses. He was fairly agile on the lower rings of the "monkey bars," but he was afraid of high places. His manipulative skills improved.

During the summer of 1970, Pedro's teacher included him two to three times a week, for an hour, in a group of two or three children. At this time, Maria, who was then two years old, began to join Pedro in the nursery. Both children, during this period, seemed depressed, withdrawn and only slightly verbal. Appointments were made for Pedro in the speech clinic, but they were not kept.

During the fall of 1970, when Maria had officially joined the group, the teachers became aware that Pedro and Maria had a special language. It was not Spanish, but a language that the children used at home and at school which no one else, even their mother, could understand. Pedro seemed exceedingly jealous of Maria's play with others in the class, especially with the boys. He was very demanding and bossy with Maria. In the meantime, Mrs. M. alternated between periods of well-being, depression and withdrawal. Mr. M. had been out of the home this time since the beginning of the year. His infrequent reappearances were the signals for serious parental battles.

In March, 1971, the Therapeutic Nursery moved out of the hospital to a community church basement. In this place, away from the hospital, most of the children in the nursery seemed to make important gains. Pedro and Maria gave up their special language. They showed greater interest in other children. At this time, three mornings a week, after the regular nursery program, the M. children had half-hour speech sessions with their own teachers. Positive results included an increase in spoken language, pointing and naming things, and using short sentences. Both children seemed to have a preference for English, and acted as if they did not understand Spanish when it was spoken by the one Spanish-speaking teacher or their mother.

Pedro had increasingly better contact with adults and children. He would run wildly into the nursery classroom, shout "Hi," and give the teacher a wild embrace. He began aggressively to defend "his property" and his rights. His attention span in self-directed activities increased. He seemed less preoccupied and more tolerant of being messy. He would initiate conversation, seek attention and pursue other children. He was better able to complete an activity, and responded to praise and encouragement. More confident in all areas, he gradually began to attempt new tasks. There were still periods, however, of withdrawal, hyperactivity, hiding and running away.

During the summer of 1971, both children attended daycamp-type sessions twice weekly for four hours each. During the bus trip to the camp, Pedro was able to name the things along the way that he recognized, and would ask "What's that?" when things were unfamiliar. He had reached his optimal level in the nursery. During this period he was being interviewed at Psychiatric Institute and had numerous contacts with his father as well as his mother. The latter joined him in interviews with the psychiatrist at the hospital. He was prepared for all of these contacts through play sessions with his teachers.

One of Mrs. M.'s initial complaints had to do with Pedro's poor eating habits. Throughout his nursery life, Pedro ate snacks with the children only sporadically. He would typically drink the juice, and sometimes sample the food other children had on their plates. However, he greatly enjoyed cake, especially birthday-party frosted cake and ice cream; during such parties he would sing "Happy birthday to you" over and over again with the others. During his final summer in the nursery, he ate small amounts of food more freely, even tasting things that were unfamiliar. Mrs. M. would often bring a lunch of spaghetti and franks from the local luncheonette. One day, however, she brought mashed potatoes with a fried egg on top, which she had herself prepared. This recalled a lunch which Mrs. M.'s mother had prepared for her in her childhood.

Psychological Evaluations and Observations

The following psychological evaluations and observations were made in June, 1969, May, 1970 and June, 1971. The first two were part of the screening process, and the other two were progress assessments. Pedro was two years and eleven months old when first seen; three years and ten months old in 1970; and four years and eleven months old in 1971.

Observation I

Pedro looked handsome and bright eyed, but quite self-absorbed, as he paced up and down with an erect gait, all by himself, in the clinic hall. Psychologist and psychiatrist saw him jointly in this screening session. Although Pedro frequently smiled, his face appeared masklike, and did not seem to reflect real feelings of pleasure. Most often, he seemed to hear and comprehend English words; however, he often ignored what was said to him and seemed to do only what *he* wanted to do. He moved vigorously and quickly, often bumping into obstacles; losing his balance, he would then slip and fall to the floor. He got up instantly, however, without looking at anybody, making a sound, or appearing shaken. He seemed not to expect help or comfort, and to inhibit anxious and painful feelings. He did not initiate contacts or make demands.

Pedro's use of pegboards was most unusual for someone barely three years old. He neither fumbled or tried to force the pegs into their holes, but proceeded in a systematic, thoughtful manner. He first surveyed a board, then aligned the pegs carefully with the edge of the holes, and in the case of the more difficult square pegs, adjusted them to make smooth insertion possible. He worked with much absorption, and was serious and tense. He evoked the image of an "absent-minded little professor." From this performance, it could be inferred that Pedro possessed some awareness of spatial relations, ability to persist in the pursuit of a goal and an unusually long attention span. A preference for the right hand was apparent, although at times he used either right or left, as is quite common at this age. Complete laterality testing to determine dominance between the right and left sides of the boy was never achieved because of his unwillingness to respond to instructions. Pedro showed curiosity toward unfamiliar objects and activities, but he would not perform when urged, even though there were indications that he could learn quickly from observations. He did not know what to do with paper and pencil, but learned how to hold a pencil and then refused to use it.

Observation II

The main product of Pedro's deprivation seemed to be great curiosity. His curiosity during a one-to-one session shortly after the first screening was well-nigh boundless. He wanted to reach everything hidden behind doors, and invaded the contents of boxes, drawers and closets. He seemed to spare no effort in satisfying this "thirst," and climbed on a chair to lift down a case of test materials from a shelf. He probed and investigated unfamiliar things with evident interest, but seemed too timid to attempt to play with them. On the other hand, when he found a familiar object, like a car or airplane, he would play with it for long periods of time, apparently completely oblivious of the observer. Occasionally he would hum while occupied in play. Once while rummaging through a carton of toys, he looked intently at a rubber figure. When asked what it was, he clearly and correctly said, "boy." This response seemed to indicate a true capacity for speech, and held some significance in terms of his self-image. On another occasion he spontaneously said, "Gimme," pointing to a car he wanted.

Pedro's ability to stack graduated wooden rings, unaided, in ascending order on a pole, represented "size discrimination" expected on a three-and-one-half-year-old level. While resistance to instructions interfered with the use of a similar but standardized test, Pedro in this instance clearly showed average ability. It was of interest that Pedro looked directly at the examiner during this session, and even stared at her.

Observation III

A year later Pedro's facial expressions were more "natural," and there were signs of greater awareness of and relatedness to another person. He greeted the observer with a fleeting smile and had a mischievous look while hiding small objects and waiting for a response. He crawled inside a large metal closet and closed the doors from the inside, a difficult task. He seemed to be testing the observer's attention and concern, and when the doors were opened and he was "discovered," his sheepish smile on emerging seemed to indicate genuine pleasure, tempered by the shock of an anxiety-provoking experience. This time he revealed a fascination with mechanical devices and an excellent skill in manipulating them. He turned the crank of a "barking" toy dog in a basket, and fixed a zipper that was stuck. Physical stamina was apparent when he carried a large heavy case across the room. He did not use intelligible language for communication, but responded to his name and was somewhat more amenable to instructions. While making eye-contact, he had involuntary, jerky head motions, which could have been manifestations of either tension and/or of minimal organic dysfunctioning. When he heard the sound of a siren, he dashed in the direction of the stimulus, and uttered explosive, garbled sounds, some of which seemed to resemble Spanish words.

When he was relaxed, he would perform an activity such as playing with an airplane to the accompaniment of a loud, possibly aggressive, consonant blend, using his lips. He still avoided any manipulation of and response to materials which were either concrete or symbolic representations of human beings, such as dolls and pictures of people. He did not at this time object to physical contact with the observer. Indeed, he retreated to her when his mother arrived to pick him up. This time he even preferred the female observer to the male psychologist whom he had earlier used for comfort and with whom he had shared his feelings during his accident. His negative response to the male psychologist followed on the heels of a fight between his parents in which Pedro had seen his mother hurt. He seemed to identify the male psychologist with his aggressive father.

Observation IV

Pedro was seen for the last time in an unfamiliar setting, but in the presence of the Spanish-speaking nursery teacher who had been his primary caretaker. He immediately made contact with the observer, taking her hand and smiling in what appeared to be a seductive manner. He was given a standardized test that required no verbal instruction and responses, even though, in the nursery, he had been speaking more often than in earlier times. Pedro employed spontaneous speech to express a wish or demand, and he would talk sporadically, primarily to draw attention to what he was doing and observing.

His repertoire of nouns was very slight, but he could speak in short, simple, functional phrases. He said, "Hello, what's that?" into a telephone; "there go car"; "look at that"; "no good"; "come on"; "get that open." While he still strenuously resisted verbal requests to imitate or respond with language, he could be drawn into nonverbal performance tasks. He would desist in a task when coaxed, but resumed voluntarily when not pressured, especially if the task seemed to appeal to him. Pedro would call out "Hi" whenever a stranger passed the room, and then would return to what he was doing. This was a stereotyped response to strangers, suggesting that his motivation was either to attract attention to himself, or that he was mechanically applying what he had learned to do when perceiving people. Once, when he was actually addressed, he appeared quite startled. In this context, it seemed highly relevant that, on a picture-completion test, Pedro was successful in handling abstract forms but failed at the same level of difficulty when the picture involved a person. His fear of people seemed deeply rooted. Notwithstanding these fears, he had begun to behave more aggressively in face-to-face contact with familiar persons.

Despite Pedro's earlier skill in manual manipulations and his perceptiveness, there were now clearer signs of difficulty with fine visual-motor coordination. This seemed to be due either to a developmental lag, or to minimal cerebral dysfunctioning. He could not reproduce a simple block design, and on the completion test reversal errors were noted. In addition, he attempted to force blocks into their stalls. When he tried to copy a circle, manual control was unsteady and weak.

The results of the examination indicated that Pedro functioned on a low average level of intelligence. His IQ on the Leiter International Performance Scale was 80, and his mental age was three years and eleven months, *i.e.* one year below his chronological age. His basal age was at the three year level, and he passed two items at age four. A ceiling was not established because of Pedro's increasing restlessness and negativism. The clinical impression, formed during the first screening contact, of greater, probably bright normal, potentialities seemed supported by the progress that has been described.

Especially in the first three observations, the examiner did not attempt a full evaluation of Pedro. This screening process provided for an approximation, a discovery of what was important in his functioning. Hypotheses concerning strengths and weaknesses were made, and evidence to confirm or deny these hypotheses was sought in various other situations. The situations were informal, and not standardized, but the examiner's experience, particularly with standardized instruments, served as control. The problems and instructions in the screening process are adapted to the needs of the child. A positive response may not be scoreable in terms of test requirements, but such responses have qualitative value inasmuch as they can indicate level of functioning. Knowledge of *range* of functioning, rather than a specific *measure*, such as an IQ, a mental age, or a developmental quotient, answers the questions "What is the best the child can do?" and "What are his potentialities?" Attempts are always made to achieve insights into thought processes, and to use these insights in ways that facilitate learning.

Pedro: A Language Appraisal
Katrina de Hirsch, F.C.S.T.
Consultant in Language Pathology
New York Psychiatric Institute and Hospital

The linguistic growth of the child unfolds through the interaction of several factors: those from within the child himself; those related to prenatal, natal and postnatal events; and those impinging on him from the environment. The child's constitutional endowment, his inherent strengths and weaknesses—genetic, physiological, emotional and linguistic—interact with environmental forces: the affective climate of the home, the quality of mothering he receives, and his social and cultural milieu.

To look at any single variable as the "cause" of a severe language deficit is to take a simplistic view. In practically every case, one has to search for the complex interactions among variables.

Pedro's massive communicative difficulties are heavily overdetermined. I believe that his communication problems stem from an organic source; his history supports this view. In an already constitutionally vulnerable youngster, the lack of good nurturing, the absence of a dependable love object, the many traumas and vicissitudes of his life must have interfered dramatically with growth in all areas, and more specifically, must have compounded his severe linguistic deficits.

The potential for language is laid down in the central nervous system. That potential is realized in the matrix of the affective and linguistic interaction between the child and his mother, who stimulates his vocalizations in situations which are comforting and pleasurable. The mother caresses the baby with her voice, and her vocalizations are tailored to his affective needs. Pedro must have missed the happy babbling conversations and the vocal play which we believe are important both to later listening attitudes and to the drive toward communication.

How do children learn to understand symbolic language? The question is highly pertinent in Pedro's case:

Children respond first to situations, and to the prosodic features of communication—pitch, intonation, inflection—which carry the emotional load of language. As they mature and their neurological organization becomes more differentiated, phonemic patterns become intertwined with prosodic features until they take dominance, regardless of the situation.

In order to comprehend, the child must make some sense out of the world that surrounds him; Pedro's world was forever shifting. He must have a rudimentary sense of self, of being separate. His central processing mechanism must be intact. Recent research shows that crude sorting and organizing of linguistic signals occurs far earlier than we knew. During the seemingly passive listening periods, the baby learns to detect certain regularities in the language that impinges on him. He begins to order the "buzzing confusion" that surrounds him into more or less stable categories. This process is of course infinitely more difficult for children who are exposed to two languages.

Pedro has failed in this respect. At this late stage, he presents a severe input disorder with comprehension difficulties that are more massive than they seem to be on first meeting with him. He fully understands situations, intonations, and all, or most, nonsymbolic cues. He also understands nouns, although he may cheerfully give one a button if one asks for the boat, or a hairbrush instead of the scissors, if the situation does not clarify the demand. He understands some verbs; he learned "jump" the other day during play. Actually, he does better with short chunks of speech than with words in isolation. But he processes only the most primitive linguistic units, and he does not begin to understand the difference between "the dog chases the boy" and "the boy chases the dog;" the order of words, which is an important linguistic signal in English, has no meaning for him. Very occasionally he interprets something more complex when it is part of a highly cathected or familiar situation.

It is, of course, true that Pedro's not-understanding is related to not-listening, which is one way of controlling the interpersonal situation, and part of his particular brand of negativism. (It is hard to say whether his early refusal to swallow was neurogenically based, or an expression of conflict in the oral area.) At any rate, not-listening serves to shut out people, and Pedro has good reason to do that. I believe that the jargon he used with his sister had, at least in part, a similar function. Actually, it would be of considerable interest to listen to their communication now; it appears that she also has language difficulties.

While the mechanism of not-listening clearly serves Pedro in some way, it is also easy for him to use because he does have severe and legitimate processing difficulties. These are compounded by exposure to two languages. Having to decode and encode in two different linguistic systems constitutes an enormous burden for children like Pedro.

This boy's input disorder is reflected in the quality of his output. His voice is quite monotonous. In some youngsters this reflects a lack of communicative intent, but monotonous speech is also heard frequently in children with central nervous system dysfunctions. His articulation is not too bad when he repeats what is said to him; when we first saw him there was some degree of echolalia. In spontaneous vocalizations, when he had the additional task of formulating even very limited content, his articulation is far less acceptable. Pedro has quite a repertoire of phrases and he adds new ones daily. Most of them are appropriate to the situation, but many are nevertheless stockphrases: "lemme see," "loo a da" (look at that), "wha da," "da boa" (that's a boat), etc. We have only seen him for three weeks, and he probably had regressed when he first entered Psychiatric Institute, but it is clear that he responds to teaching. He now generates much more language. When he gets wrapped up in train play, which obviously plays an important part in his fantasies, he articulates fewer words and sounds much more diffuse. When the therapist manages to engage him in different activities, which was at first quite difficult, his verbal output has a much more socialized quality.

Like most language-deprived children, Pedro is very concrete. For example, he will sit himself on the toy toilet. In other words, he does not quite comprehend the representational character of toys. What concerns me is the paucity of inner language, and the fact that Pedro does not use language sufficiently to mediate tasks.

There have been many positive changes. Pedro now shows some interest in human figure drawing, and he has lately used doll figures extensively in his play, which has become much more dramatic. We do not provide any interpretations; it is not our role to play out conflictual material. But the affect aroused during this kind of play is essential in stimulating language production.

I feel sure that the Therapeutic Nursery at Harlem Hospital has saved Pedro, psychologically. He does, now, have a measure of trust in the adult, and he does make efforts to relate beyond the need-fulfilling level.

Children such as Pedro, however, should be exposed to intensive language stimulation early, between 24 and 30 months. At later ages, the "critical" period, that time when the organism is most sensitive to specific kinds of stimulation, may have passed. There is a biological and psychological timetable for language, and I firmly believe that at later stages, when the brain is less plastic, it is far harder to help children process input and activate output. And I am absolutely sure that severe processing difficulties at age three are the precursors of massive learning disorders.

How does one work with language-delayed children? To begin with, it is essential to cut out the second language. I fully realize that this is not something one undertakes lightly. The goal for most dual-culture children is to enable them to participate in both cultures—their own and that of the mainstream of the society. Cutting a child off from his "mother" language has many psychological and sociological implications. Nevertheless, in children such as Pedro one has no choice.

It may be appropriate to discuss briefly some approaches to language stimulation. There are some which are counterproductive. One does not ever ask a child to repeat words or phrases. One does not tell him, "Say this or say that." Once speech becomes part of the child's negativistic pattern, one is beaten before one starts. One does not correct the articulation of a child; correction extinguishes communication. One does not present them with pictures and objects and say, "This is a fish" or "a boat" or what have you. The referential function of language has little to do with communication.

Learning in young children must be infused with the energy derived from their drives and affects. Therefore, speech is acquired as an outflow of highly cathected situations in the framework of a close relationship with the therapist and the people who care for the child, hopefully for very extended periods of time.

We have drawn up an intensive language stimulation program for Pedro, and we have the help of the ward and teaching staff. Modeling is the therapy of choice. We accompany what Pedro does with short model verbalizations which fit into his needs of the moment. We expand what he says into slightly longer linguistic units. We literally feed him phrases and short sentences during play. If he hits himself, the therapist puts her arms around him and says, "Poor Pedro, it hurts; look at that sharp corner." This teaches him three new concepts as part of an emotionally loaded situation: empathy, the recognition and acceptance of pain, the meaning of "sharp corner." In this kind of learning, cognitive and affective streams flow together.

Prognosis for Pedro is guarded. I believe that he will make highly significant strides in spoken language, which will make all the difference in terms of his becoming a functioning member of society. But I am not sure what the goals should be in terms of education. I do not as yet know what his potential for abstraction is. And I do not know as yet how he will cope with second order verbal symbols; that is, with printed language.

Furthermore, it is not yet clear how far Pedro's linguistic deficits have interfered with ego development. Anna Freud (1936) has said:

> The attempt to take hold of the drive processes by linking them with verbal signs which can be dealt with in consciousness is one of the most general, earliest and most necessary accomplishments of the human ego. We regard it as an indispensable component of the ego, not as one among its activities [p. 461].

Improved language tools can be expected to reduce Pedro's hyperactivity and assist impulse control. Ability to express his feelings will alleviate some of his severe anxieties and fears.

At best the road will be long and arduous.

Summary

Nature, nurture, and noxia all play outstanding roles in the lives of many developing infants and children in the Harlem Hospital Center community. Pedro was not unusual in this regard. Pedro's presence at Psychiatric Institute, as well as his two years' stay in the Developmental Unit of the Division of Child Psychiatry, represents the interdisciplinary team's recognition of Pedro's ego strength; its survival value and its adaptive capabilities in the face of possible constitutional deficits, inadequate nurturing and outstanding trauma. The presence of ego strength, wherever it is found, demands our active, on-the-spot support, and the best that we have in the way of remedies. If we are fortunate enough to assist Pedro in reassembling his ego building-blocks; if we can discover how he has survived in the face of damage, deficit and trauma; and should we find ourselves able to suit our remedies to his needs; then our knowledge of development, normal and abnormal, of protective mechanisms in the process of development that is "off course," and of ways to adapt old treatment modes to the needs of all of our population, including the most advantaged as well as the most deprived, will be immeasurably enhanced.

In Pedro's case, a diagnosis of constitutional deficit due to accidental injury and medication during his mother's pregnancy was at best equivocal. However, lack of speech, poor coordination, including visuo-motor coordination, and lack of balance pointed to possible minimal cerebral dysfunction.

Pedro was born into a family in which the mother's great dependency needs were the product of the loss through death of her own mother when she was twelve; the loss of her father through his remarriage; and the loss of her native home when her family moved to New York. Her feelings of dependency were increased by separation from her husband and the death of the grandmother who had reared her. She had, however, spent one year in college and may be a creative writer. The background of Pedro's father is less well known to us. He is, no doubt, temperamentally aggressive. He and Pedro's mother give evidence of at least average intellectual ability.

Pedro's mother's dependency needs and narcissism were remarkable. We were saddened and amused by the frequent sight of three-or four-year-old Pedro, walking several paces in front of his mother, his back ramrod straight, a smirk on his face, his hands in his pockets, advancing in a "slew-footed" fashion. As described by Anna Freud (1965), he evinced "exaggerated manliness" and "noisy aggression"; that is, "overcompensations which betray underlying castration fears." Pedro, who was capable of this defensive maneuver, had sufficient ego-strength to "pull it off." On another occasion, at home, when he witnessed a sexual battle between his parents, a "primal scene," Pedro was, in reality, called upon by his mother to protect her. Following this traumatic incident, in his play with family dolls, he indicated his ambivalence. He wanted to be at his father's side and to be identified with his father's aggressiveness.

Pedro had profound conflicts on almost every level of development. He was able to compensate for some of these difficulties and interferences. He spat out his food as early as two months of age, and remained a "feeding problem" from that time on. He gained weight, however. In Erikson's terms, he was "unable to trust," and even avoided representations of people. He was, however, able to make fairly good object relationships in spite of the fact that television had been his early caretaker, and he always maintained at least nonverbal communication with adults. He preferred men to women, and could expose his feelings to the former. He learned to toilet himself on his own at two, conforming to the wishes of his mother. He also indicated trouble at the anal level by his avoidance of messiness. His own aggressiveness, as well as that of the men with whom he identified, frightened him. He was conflicted in the aggressive use of his mouth for speech and chewing. On the other hand, an aggressive negativism both inhibited his functioning, and protected him from the onslaughts of the environment.

Pedro's relationship with his sister was both rivalrous, and mutually supportive. This was further evidence of his good object relationships. By the age of three, he appeared capable of internalizing his agressive feelings, exchanging them for self-destructive behavior. He was finally able to accept loving concern from men and women. With his improved ability to corroborate and validate feelings of fear, pain and affection, his self-image improved. He knew himself as "one who is loved."

Pedro regressed repeatedly in response to physical and emotional trauma, and in response to his mother's exaggerated dependency needs. He made gains in object relationships, speech and other behavior, in an environment supportive to him and his family. Members of a clinical-educational team actively provided opportunities for Pedro to perceive himself in a positive light, and to fully accept his own feelings. Therapeutic education and on-the-spot catharsis and other brief therapies were the chief modes of treatment. Categorizing Pedro diagnostically would seem to have doubtful value. Pedro is not a psychotic child.

Pedro, at five years of age, still requires a more consistent, less injurious environment than he has had in the past. A residential treatment and educational setting was indicated. This is a crucial time in Pedro's development, with particular reference to speech. In July, 1971, Pedro was referred to the Psychiatric Institute.

This work with Pedro and his family has demanded a well-coordinated team approach. The above report was prepared by all members of the team. We are grateful for the assistance and support of Dr. Virginia Wilking, Chief of the Division of Child Psychiatry, and Dr. Elizabeth B. Davis, Director of the Department of Psychiatry, Harlem Hospital Center. We are also grateful for the continued help of our colleagues at the New York State Psychiatric Institute, who now serve Pedro and his family.

Frances Gautieri Ricigliano, A.C.S.W., Formerly Senior Social Worker, Developmental Psychiatry Unit, Division of Child Psychiatry

Helen R. Drew, B.S., Educational Director of the Therapeutic Nursery and Educational Consultant, Developmental Psychiatry Unit, Division of Child Psychiatry

Irene J. Spanier, M.S., Chief Psychologist, Division of Child Psychiatry

Margaret Morgan Lawrence, M.D., Attending Psychiatrist, Developmental Psychiatry Unit, Division of Child Psychiatry

Harlem Hospital Center
October 1971

VII

MISSION

> With the emergence of the Community Mental Health movement, many professionals are adopting a different perspective, which suggests that limited therapeutic resources must be deployed in such a manner as to inject change-inducing elements into faulty family and social systems as early as possible [Barten & Barten, 1973, p. 3].

Young Inner City Families—The Development of Ego Strength Under Stress narrates some of the hazards of early child development in an urban black community. It relates the struggles of an interdisciplinary mental health team as it attempts to assess the damage to these families, their infants and young children.

The story did not begin in Harlem. It is an urban, exaggerated variant of lives lived by parents, grandparents and great-grandparents of these families, chiefly in rural Southern areas. Because of injuries in ancestral social scenes, young families are a ready prey to the more concentrated traumata of the city. These are young persons fleeing families and communities, scenes of conflicts unbearable to them, in which they had seen no hope of productive lives. The story is not a tale of unrelieved despair. Strength abounds in these families and it, too, is a reflection, to some extent, of the survival of an inherited strength by all the avenues open to inheritance: nature, nurture and culture.

The Developmental Psychiatry Unit team in this story is dominated, and ofttimes even propelled to energetic on-the-spot action, by the knowledge that the dynamics of development, the role of the unconscious, the possibilities for insight and the existence of a true feeling life cannot be denied in the poor and the black. Change in behavior, for the better—knowledgeably tapped by persons committed to the humanity of the people with whom they work, and with a lively expectation of positive response on the part of latent ego strengths—does occur. Psychodynamic insight even lends itself to "impulse control."

A 24-year-old mother began to cuff her frail looking four-year-old boy when she would meet him at the end of the nursery day. She seemed oblivious of the observing teachers. This boy was the family's second son. During his first six months in the nursery he had been conforming and provocative in turn. Although the mother and father had participated in a thoroughgoing intake study, as well as family visits and parent meetings, the new flavor of "child abuse" in the mother-son relationship prompted a review of this family's story.

It was not easy to find these six family members at home at any one time. Usually the mother denied that it was possible for her husband to be at home with her and the children when a team member would make a family visit. However, urged on by our nursery child's need, we made a number of contacts with both parents which did finally result in the presence of mother, father and the two younger children during a family visit with a psychiatrist and social worker from the unit team. We sat closely but comfortably in a small room, furnished with several folded cots and a table, which was separated from the parental bedroom only by a long bookcase; above the bookcase hung strings of brightly colored beads. The tiny apartment was furnished with good taste and imagination. It was the first time that I had seen the mother's "beauty school" diploma on the wall; and while the mother was preparing cups of coffee, the father showed us pictures in their family album. The family had just come from an island in the Caribbean the year before, and the father was proudly showing pictures of the two older children, in costume, in a Mardi Gras parade. The father said that he himself had made the children's costumes, and that they had won first prize. We were duly impressed and said so.

When the adults were again all present in the room, one of the unit team asked, "Who does Tony, your four-year old, remind you of?" "He's just like my younger brother," the mother responded impatiently. "My mother made me take care of him. I was seventeen then, married, and had my own child. He was weak, had asthma. When she wasn't there, he would make me so angry that I would hit him." "I remember," added the father, "although I was never around your mother's house much during the day. I stayed at my father's place." "You did until the time when you lost your job," said Mrs. W. Again she looked irritated and almost shouted, "You suddenly took a vacation in Trinidad, for six months, just after I became pregnant with Tony. You wanted me to come to Trinidad, too, but my mother wouldn't let me because I was pregnant. Tony was born and you were still away. My mother said then that the baby was too small to travel. Tony was six months old before the two children and I got to Trinidad. Come to think of it, Tony *is* like my brother."

"You're always hitting on Tony," the father challenged. "Yeah," mused Mrs. W. "I think every time I look at Tony I get mad, exactly like I used to feel when I would look at my brother." "And," Mr. W. said, "I feel like taking up for Tony because you and the big one always pick on him. I know how he feels."

Mrs. W. was warm, hardworking and intelligent. We believe that parental insights helped to save Tony from further abuse. Free acceptance of feelings in an atmosphere of mutual respect provided opportunities for insight, emotional re-education and change in behavior. In some mental health circles, this approach is met with opposition; it is believed that catharsis of "dated emotions" in treatment requires extensive preparation and preliminary establishment of rapport. Our response to this argument, supported by this book's narrative, is that effective dynamically oriented education and treatment can be provided in a relatively short time, and in other than orthodox circumstances, under conditions of openness, respect and trust. The mental health worker needs, together with a humanizing attitude, self-knowledge and self-discipline that does not permit exploitation of the poor, the black, or a child. With mutual respect and self-knowledge on the part of the therapist, a common humanity will reveal itself. It may well be that it is the "advantaged" person's lack of openness and fear of exposure that makes the less-advantaged person appear flat, distant and unavailable to insight. Consultation, from a psychodynamic orientation, with other professionals and paraprofessionals in education and health has schooled me in this approach, more than any other experience. I would agree that not all families with multiple problems will respond; many do, and their numbers are sufficient to demand such exploration.

When the hazards of the Harlem community impair "nature" among our infants and young children, our team of workers tries to foster more and better communication between the damaged child and the adults significant to him. We offer our tools to young families under our care and to other agencies which also serve them, so that families may know their own gifts for "nurturing" their children. Our work with other agencies is both consultative and collaborative, and whenever possible we share with them efforts toward the betterment of the community's living conditions. Similarly, we educate and support families in providing settings free from overwhelming traumatic influences.

We propose action-oriented, on-the-spot training and experience for prospective child psychiatrists and pediatricians, for graduate students in clinical psychology, speech and language therapy, psychiatric nursing and psychiatric social work. Persons who are concerned with the problems of child development in the context of the urban family and community, and who intend to pursue their concern by joining an interdisciplinary mental health team such as our own, should have their training and experience in such teams. Paraprofessionals who come from the Harlem community share the work of our Developmental Psychiatry Unit team. They are hard-working, insightful, talented persons, whom we have chosen for these gifts. They contribute fully as team members in conferences, clinics, nurseries and homes, and are important communication factors among them all. When a mother of five children, one of whom was a child in our nursery, became suicidal and had to be hospitalized, the nursery's long-time transportation aide and teacher assistant went to the children that day in their home. She remained there overnight, and for 24 hours, until a relative could be summoned from another borough. Her duties included the care of two-year-old twin boys and the support of a frightened adolescent boy. She did not work alone, but in close contact with teachers, social workers, psychiatrists, relatives and the Department of Welfare. There was no "overtime" pay in the budget with which to reward her. Members of teams in training can profit by exposure to a human being like this one.

Our approach to the poor and the black is no substitute for necessary basic social change. I am repeatedly reminded by members of the younger generations that important changes must be made in a society which offers so many hazards to the growth, development, safety and future of so many of its people. This would seem to indicate, if this premise is accepted, that persons trained in the mental health disciplines are bound to work to some extent on two fronts: the one for which their disciplines have specifically prepared them, and the other to be shared with larger segments of the community, a front that is dedicated to fundamental social change. Respect and dynamic understanding of individuals, their strengths and needs, informs social approaches. Awareness of community needs enriches our support of the strength of individuals. Will the strengths of young Harlem families survive until significant changes in hazardous social patterns and institutions occur? We are committed to this faith, and from it derive our hope.

REFERENCES

Barten, H. H. & Barten, S. S. New perspectives in child mental health. In H. H. Barten & S. S. Barten (Eds.), *Children and their parents in brief therapy*. New York: Behavioral Publications, 1973.

Bernard, V. W. Composite remedies for psychosocial problems. In G. Belasso (Ed.), Psychiatric care of the underprivileged. Vol. 8. *International psychiatry clinics*. Boston: Little, Brown and Company, 1971, 8 (2), 61–85.

Bowlby, J. Attachment and loss. Vol. 1. *Attachment*. New York: Basic Books, 1969.

Erikson, E. H. Ego development and historical change. *Identity and the life cycle* (Psychological Issues 1). New York: International Universities Press, 1959, 18–49.

Erikson, E. H. Growth and crises of the healthy personality. *Identity and the life cycle* (Psychological Issues 1). New York: International Universities Press, 1959, 50–100.

Escalona, S. K. *The roots of individuality*. Chicago: Aldine, 1968.

Freud, A. *Ego and the mechanism of defense.* 1936. Tr. by L. Peller. New York: International Universities Press, 1946, 178. Cited by L. Peller, *Psycho-analytic study of the child.* Vol. XXI. New York: International Universities Press, 1966, 461.

Freud, A. Normality and pathology in childhood: assessments of development. Vol. VI. *The writings of Anna Freud.* New York: International Universities Press, 1965.

Jones, B. E., Lightfoot, O. B., Palmer, D., Wilkerson, R. G., & Williams, D. H. Problems of black psychiatric residents in white training institutes. *American Journal of Psychiatry,* December, 1970, **127,** 798–803.

Knoblock, H. & Pasamanick, B. Further observations on the behavioral development of Negro children. *The Journal of Genetic Psychology,* 1953, **83,** 137–157.

Kolb, L. C. The concept of the community mental health center. In L. C. Kolb, V. W. Bernard, B. P. Dohrenwend (Eds.), *Urban challenges to psychiatry.* Boston: Little, Brown and Company, 1969.

Lawrence, C. R. The psychoanalyst and community mental health. Verbal statement made during the workshop at the meeting of the American Academy of Psychoanalysis, New Orleans, December, 1968.

Lawrence, M. M. *Mental health team in the schools.* New York: Behavioral Publications, 1971.

Lilienfeld, A. M. & Pasamanick, B. Association of maternal and fetal factors with the development of mental deficiency. *American Journal of Mental Deficiency.* January, 1956, **60**, 557–569.

Murray, P. To the oppressors (poem). In *Dark testament.* Norwalk, Conn.: Silvermine, 1970.

O'Gorman, N. *The wilderness and the laurel tree.* New York: Harper and Row, 1972.

Prudhomme, C. Reflections on racism. *American Journal of Psychiatry,* December, 1970, **127**, 815–7.

Report of the Joint Commission on Mental Health of Children. *Crisis in child mental health: challenge for the 1970's.* New York: Harper and Row, 1969.

Report to Governor Nelson A. Rockefeller by the New York State Committee for Children. *A child advocacy system in New York State.* New York, 1971.

Spiegel, J. Position statement for the annual presidential election. American Psychiatric Association, Spring, 1973.

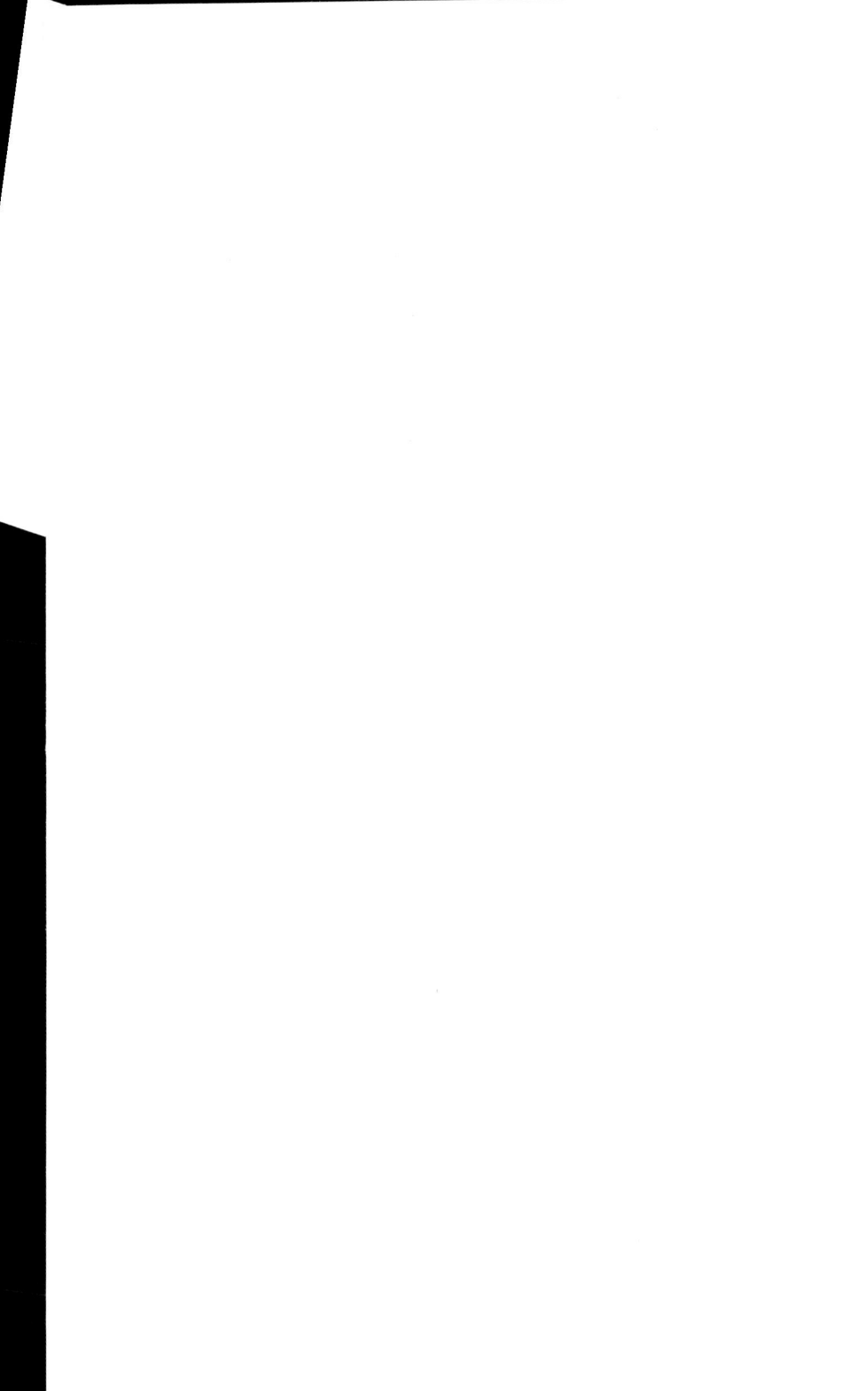

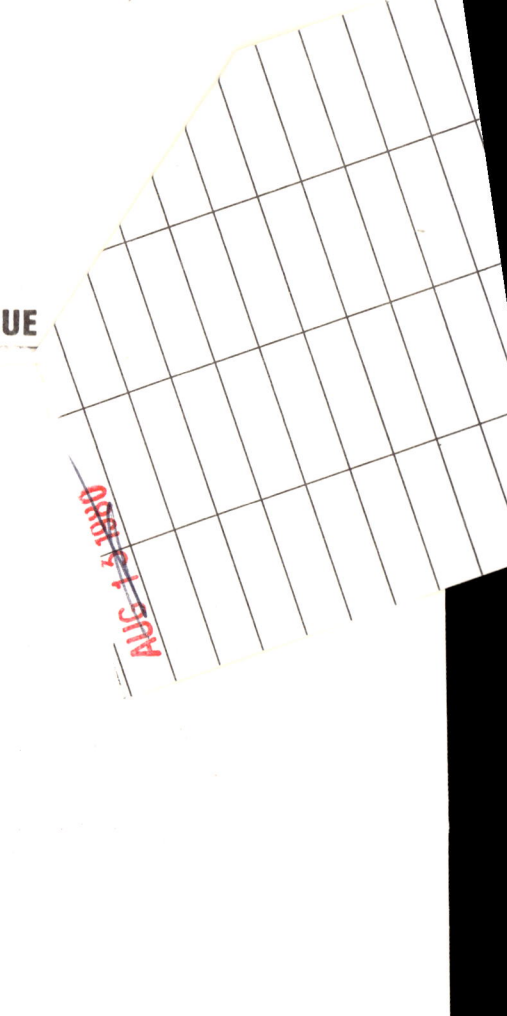